EXERCISES FOR WOMEN

EXERCISES FOR WOMEN*

RIVKA GADISH

* who suffer from urine leakage, lack of libido,
and impaired vitality.

Astrolog ◆ The Quality of Life Series ◆

Series editor: Sara Bleich
Editor: Marion Duman
Cover design: Na'ama Yaffe
Layout and Graphics: Ruth Erez
Production Manager: Dan Gold
Photographs applied by the author.

ISBN 965-494-118-X

Published by Astrolog Publishing House 2001

Astrolog Publishing House

P. O. Box 1123, Hod Hasharon 45111, Israel
Tel: 972-9-7412044
Fax: 972-9-7442714
E-Mail: info@astrolog.co.il

Printed in Israel

1 3 5 7 9 10 8 6 4 2

Introduction

The method presented in this book cosists of sets of exercises that are performed lying on your back or on your stomach, sitting on a chair, and standing. All you need to start the session is comfortable clothing, two large and two small balls, uncluttered space, and about twenty minutes to devote to yourself and your health.

First you must learn all the exercises, day by day, according to the program. Then you can choose the exercises that suit you, your fitness level, and your time-frame.

During the first week, you must learn the principles that recur in all the exercises (1-7). After learning them, you do not repeat the exercises of the first week, but integrate them into all the exercises.

After you acquirethe principles, there are the sets of exercises.

The first set: Second week: First day - exercises 1-15. This set is performed on one day, and the exercises are, in fact, the most basic ones that are done (later on) in every session. This set of exercises is performed lying on your back, and takes about 15 minutes.

The second set: Second week: Second day - exercises 1-10. This set is performed on one day, lying on your back.

The third set: Second week: Third day - one special exercise that deals with the body's asymmetry.

The fourth set: Second week: Fourth day - exercises 1-6. This set is performed lying on your side.

The fifth set: Second week: Fifth day - exercises 1-6. This set is performed lying on your stomach.

The sixth set: Second week: Sixth day - exercises 1-18. This set is performed sitting on a chair. (Note the easier alternative way of performing the exercise.)

The seventh set: Second week: Seventh day - exercises 1-12 or 1-8 with two balls. This set is performed standing up, with two alternatives.

The eighth set: Second week: Three strengthening exercises for women who are very fit.

As was mentioned before, learning the sets of exercises is the first stage. Try to learn them in two weeks, even though the second week will be difficult and full. On each day of the second week, do one set only. If you do not succeed in learning the method in two weeks, take more time - for instance, two sets per week - but not more than six weeks.

After you have learned the exercise method, draw up a fixed and systematic exercise schedule, preferably once a day.

In every session, it is advisable to start with the exercises described for the first day of the second week (pages 26-55), and add another set of your choice. The additional set can be changed each day.

The length of the session is about 20 minutes. If you want to increase the level of effort, do all the sets, beginning with the basic one, through the eighth one, which is meant for women who are very fit. The full session takes about an hour.

The aim of the exercises

To strengthen and improve the female system and prevent urine leakage (incontinence).

Moreover, the exercises affect and safeguard the organism's state of health, beauty, flexibility, and strength by molding the body and improving the general state of health. This is a unique and exclusive exercise method for strengthening the female system and preventing urine leakage.

As a rule, exercise is good for everyone, but it is especially good for women of all ages. It is extremely important for post-natal women, for middle-aged women, and for third-age women.

I developed this method when I had a feminine/personal problem for which, according to the doctors, there was only a surgical solution. Performing the exercises prevented the surgery. I have disseminated this knowledge in workshops and in private treatments, and now I am writing it down.

By means of a series of targeted exercises, the pupil becomes familiar with dormant muscles and organs, and learns to use them so as to cure the diseases that are caused by the weakening or atrophying of those muscles.

The exercises are simple, natural, and non-aggressive, and follow the "everyone can" method, without age limitations. They require nothing but self-discipline.

The exercises are based on daily activation of our body systems as follows: contracting-relaxing, closing-opening. There is no need to make sharp or sudden movements.

Most of the muscles participate in the exercises, and special emphasis is placed on the unique breathing, the strengthening of the muscles of the pelvic floor, the anterior and posterior openings (urinary and anal openings), the muscles of the middle of the body and the back, the abdomen, the tongue, and the nostrils.

Learning the exercises is divided up into a detailed program (starting on page 9) of between two and six weeks.

The exercises are performed slowly, and are neither painful nor strenuous.

The importance of breathing!

The average rate of breathing is 15-16 breathing cycles (inhaling and exhaling) per minute.

With the slow breathing technique, the number of breathing cycles per minute is 5-7 (each inhaling-exhaling cycle taking about 10-12 seconds).

You have to learn how to breathe from your abdomen - filling your lungs with air to the depths of the abdominal cavity.

Inhaling is done only via the nose.

Exhaling is done by sucking the abdomen inward, and expelling the air via the mouth.

You must practice the breathing technique; it is important to understand and perform the breathing and the inward sucking of the abdomen correctly.

This exercise - the breathing and the inward sucking of the abdomen - is important and effective, and constitutes an integral part of all the exercises.

Because of the manner of breathing, the breathing becomes deeper (without the effort of running), and the blood vessels expand to allow a better flow of blood and oxygen to the muscles.

The work program

First week: first day

Learning all the organs that take part in contraction and relaxation.

Devote the first day to learning only inhaling and sucking the abdomen inward. If at first it seems difficult, don't give up - practice every day and you'll see how easy and even pleasant it becomes.

Exercise number 1:

Breathing and sucking the abdomen inward and upward using the slow technique, 5-7 breathing cycles per minute.
Lie comfortably on your back (legs bent or straight).

Relaxation (inhaling)

Inhale slowly through the nose, and fill your lungs with air right into the abdominal cavity. (Inhaling must be done slowly, taking about five seconds.)

Contraction (exhaling)

Suck the abdomen inward and pull it upward, and exhale the air through your mouth. (This action must take about two seconds.)

When the abdomen is squeezed inward, close your mouth and continue exhaling through your nose. (This action must take about 3-4 seconds.)

(Don't think about "seconds"; you should inhale the air slowly and exhale it slowly, resulting in 5-7 breathing cycles per minute.)

Relaxation (inhaling)

Inhale slowly through your nose, and fill your lungs with air right into the abdominal cavity.

The movements flow harmoniously without interrupting the breathing.

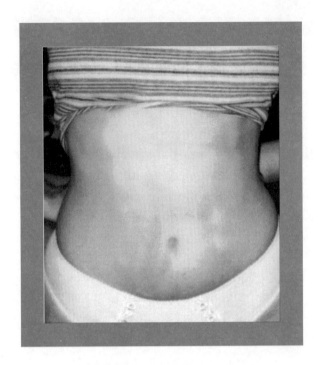

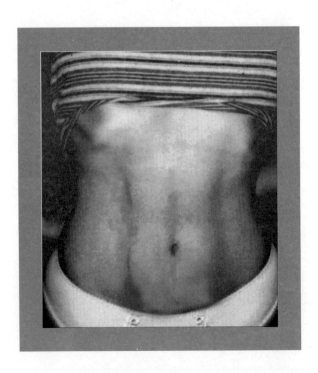

Exercises for Women

Repetition

Repeat the relaxation and contraction using the slow technique for about 20 minutes.

Devote the first day only to learning to inhale and suck the abdomen inward. Repeat the slow technique over and over again.

Don't despair if at first inhaling and sucking the abdomen inward seem to be difficult tasks. Later on, with practice, these techniques will become easy, enjoyable, and extremely healthy.

N.B.

Contraction is divided into two parts. The first is sucking the abdomen inward and upward and exhaling through the mouth. In the second, when the abdomen is squeezed inward and upward, you close your mouth, and exhale through your nose. All the contractions participate in this part.

First week: second day

Exercise number 2:

Adding the contraction of the anterior and posterior openings using the slow technique of 5-7 breathing cycles per minute.

Lie on your back with your legs bent or straight.

Relaxation (inhaling)

Inhale slowly through your nose, and fill your lungs with air right into the abdominal cavity.

Contraction (exhaling)

Suck your abdomen inward and upward and exhale through your mouth.

When your abdomen is squeezed inward, close your mouth and continue exhaling through your nose.

Clench your fists.

Now add the contraction of the anterior and posterior openings (as if you are pulling them upward into the abdominal cavity; if you neither control nor feel the anterior opening, contract the posterior opening, and in that way you will succeed in controlling the anterior opening).

Relaxation (inhaling)

Inhale slowly through your nose, and fill your lungs with air right into the abdominal cavity.

Relax the contractions (unclench your fists).

Relax the contractions of the anterior and posterior openings.

The movements flow harmoniously.

Repetition

Repeat the contraction and relaxation using the slow technique for about 20 minutes.

N.B.

All the contractions are performed together when the abdomen is sucked inward, the mouth is shut, and the air is exhaled through the nose. Breathing is smooth and uninterrupted.

It is very important to know that under no circumstances must women push and press their lower pelvis outward (as during a bowel movement), but must just contract and pull the valves upward and inward. (For men, the outward movement is permitted and desirable.)

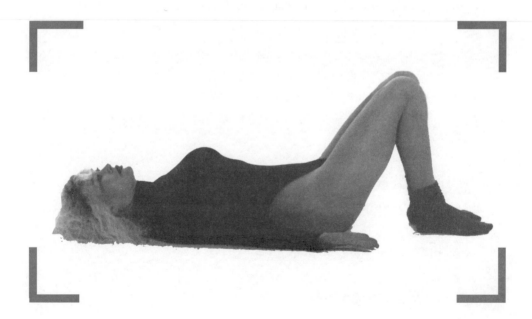

First week: third day

Exercise number 3:

Adding the contraction of the hands (clenching) using the slow technique of 5-7 breathing cycles per minute.

Lie on your back with your legs bent or straight.

Relaxation (inhaling)

Inhale slowly through your nose, and fill your lungs with air right into the abdominal cavity.

Contraction (exhaling)

Suck your abdomen inward and upward and exhale through your mouth.

When your abdomen is squeezed inward, close your mouth and continue exhaling through your nose.

While exhaling through your nose, clench your fists.

N.B.

All the contractions are performed together when the abdomen is sucked inward, the mouth is shut, and the air is exhaled through the nose.

Relaxation (inhaling)

Inhale slowly through your nose, and fill your lungs with air right into the abdominal cavity.

Relax the contractions (unclench your fists).

The movements flow harmoniously.

Repetition

Repeat the contraction and relaxation using the slow technique for about 20 minutes.

> *N.B.*
>
> *All the contractions are performed together when the abdomen is sucked inward, the mouth is shut, and the air is exhaled through the nose. Breathing is smooth and uninterrupted.*
> *It is very important to know that under no circumstances must women push and press their lower pelvis outward (as during a bowel movement), but must just contract and pull the valves upward and inward.*

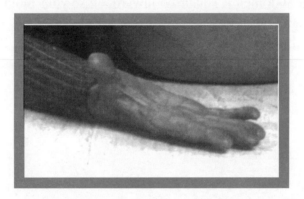

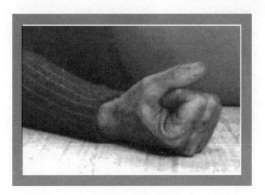

First week: fourth day

Relaxation (inhaling)

Inhale slowly through your nose, and fill your lungs with air right into the abdominal cavity.

Contraction (exhaling)

Suck your abdomen inward and upward and exhale through your mouth.

When your abdomen is squeezed inward, close your mouth and continue exhaling through your nose.

Clench your fists.

Contract your anterior and posterior openings.

To the contractions, add the pressure of your tongue on your palate. (Close your mouth and clench your teeth.)

Relaxation (inhaling)

Inhale slowly through your nose, and fill your lungs with air right into the abdominal cavity.

Relax the contractions (unclench your fists).

Relax your anterior and posterior openings.

Relax the pressure of your tongue on your hard palate.

The movements flow harmoniously.

Repetition

Repeat the relaxation and contraction using the slow technique for about 20 minutes.

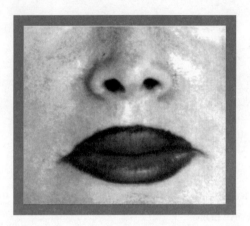

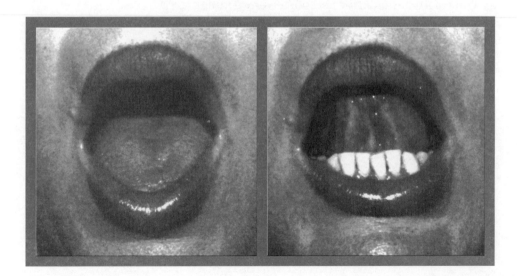

First week: fifth day

Exercise number 5:

Adding the contraction of the nostrils using the slow technique of 5-7 breathing cycles per minute.

Relaxation (inhaling)

Inhale slowly through your nose, and fill your lungs with air right into the abdominal cavity.

Contraction (exhaling)

Suck your abdomen inward and upward and exhale through your mouth.

When your abdomen is squeezed inward, close your mouth and continue exhaling through your nose.

Clench your fists.

Contract your anterior and posterior openings.

Press your tongue to your palate. (Close your mouth and clench your teeth.)

To the contractions, add the contraction of the nostrils by bringing them closer to each other.

Relaxation (inhaling)

Inhale slowly through your nose, and fill your lungs with air right into the abdominal cavity.

Relax the contractions (unclench your fists).

Relax your anterior and posterior openings.

Relax the pressure of your tongue on your palate.

Relax the contraction of your nostrils.

The movements flow harmoniously.

Repetition

Repeat the relaxation and contraction using the slow technique for about 20 minutes.

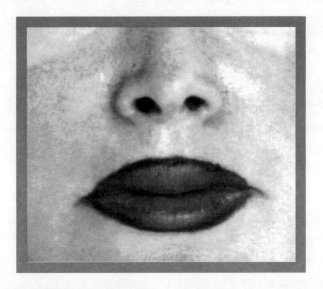

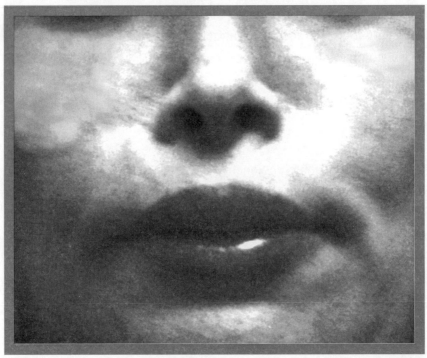

First week: sixth day

Exercise number 6:

Adding the rolling of the eyes upward (opening the eyes and pulling them upward) using the slow technique of 5-7 breathing cycles per minute.

Relaxation (inhaling)

Inhale slowly through your nose, and fill your lungs with air right into the abdominal cavity.

Contraction (exhaling)

Suck your abdomen inward and upward and exhale through your mouth.

When your abdomen is squeezed inward, close your mouth and continue exhaling through your nose.

Clench your fists.

Contract your anterior and posterior openings.

Press your tongue to your palate. (Close your mouth and clench your teeth.)

To the contractions, add the contraction of the nostrils by bringing them closer to each other.

Your eyes look upward, open (don't contract your forehead - just look upward).

Relaxation (inhaling)

Inhale slowly through your nose, and fill your lungs with air right into the abdominal cavity.

Relax the contractions (unclench your fists).

Relax your anterior and posterior openings.

Relax the pressure of your tongue on your hard palate.

Relax the contraction of your nostrils.

Release your eyes.

The movements flow harmoniously.

Repetition

Repeat the relaxation and contraction using the slow technique for about 20 minutes.

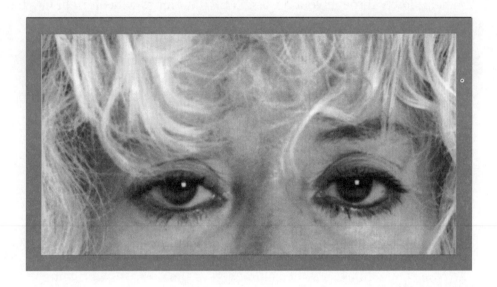

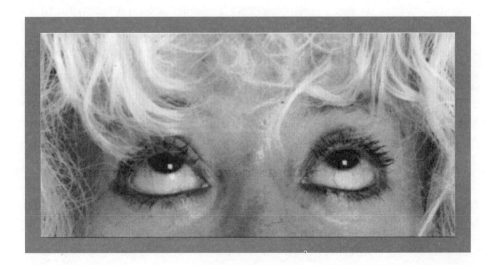

First week: seventh day

Relaxation (inhaling)

Inhale slowly through your nose, and fill your lungs with air right into the abdominal cavity.

Contraction (exhaling)

Suck your abdomen inward and upward and exhale through your mouth.

When your abdomen is squeezed inward, close your mouth and continue exhaling through your nose.

Clench your right / left fist.

Contract your anterior and posterior openings.

Press your tongue to your palate.

Contract your right / left nostril.

Your eyes look upward and to the right.

Relaxation (inhaling)

Inhale slowly through your nose, and fill your lungs with air right into the abdominal cavity.

Relax the contractions.

Contraction (exhaling)

Suck your abdomen inward and upward and exhale through your mouth.

When your abdomen is squeezed inward, close your mouth and continue exhaling through your nose.

Clench your left / right fist.

Contract your anterior and posterior openings.

Press your tongue to your palate.

Contract your left / right nostril.

Your eyes look upward and to the left.

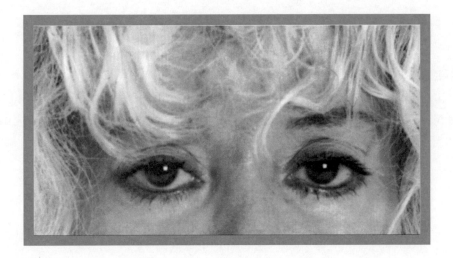

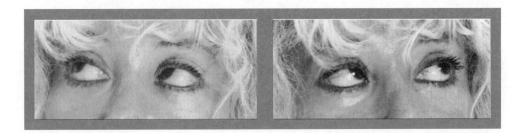

Relaxation (inhaling)

Inhale slowly through your nose, and fill your lungs with air right into the abdominal cavity.

Relax the contractions.

The movements flow harmoniously.

Repetition

Repeat the relaxation and contraction using the slow technique for about 20 minutes, contracting the right side once, and contracting the left side once.

You must learn this weekly technique.

Breathing - Relaxation - Contraction

For young women, post-partum young women, middle-aged women, and third-age women:

Discover feminine beauty
The beauty of your body
The beauty of life
Is at your feet
All you have to do is take it
Get up early, drink a cup of coffee
Find a quiet corner in your home
Inhale, relax, contract, 20 minutes
Feel what is happening inside your body
Feel that things are beginning to move
The world is opening up in front of you
You are more beautiful than ever.

During the second week, you will learn to perform the exercises using balls of different sizes. (See pictures.)

Second week: first day

Exercise number 1:

Lie on your back, legs bent, arms at the sides of your body, knees holding a ball, and each hand holding a ball. (See picture.)

Relaxation (inhaling)

Inhale slowly through your nose, and fill your lungs with air right into the abdominal cavity.

Contraction (exhaling)

Suck your abdomen inward and upward and exhale through your mouth.

When your abdomen is squeezed inward, close your mouth and continue exhaling through your nose.

While exhaling through the nose, do all the contractions:

Contract your anterior and posterior openings.

Squeeze the ball with your knees.

Squeeze the balls with your fingers.

Press your tongue to your palate (close your mouth and clench your teeth).

Contract your nostrils.

Your eyes look upward, open (don't contract your forehead; feel as if all the muscles are pulling upward in the direction of your eyes).

Relaxation (inhaling)

Inhale slowly through your nose, fill your lungs with air right into the abdominal cavity, and relax all the contractions.

The movements flow harmoniously.

Repetition

Repeat the relaxation and contraction using the slow technique about 10 times.

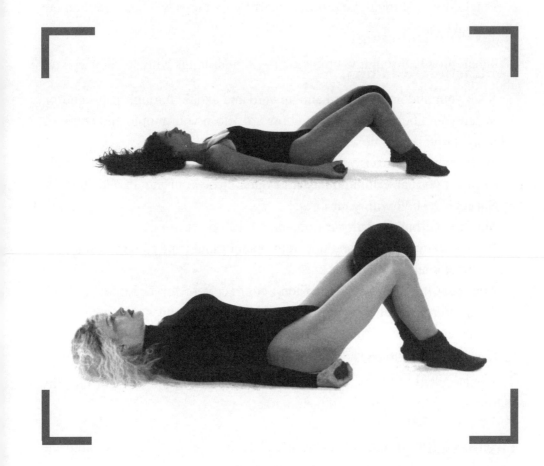

Exercise number 2:

Lie on your back, legs bent, arms straight out, knees holding a ball, and each hand holding a ball. (See picture.)

Relaxation (inhaling)

Inhale slowly through your nose, and fill your lungs with air right into the abdominal cavity.

Contraction (exhaling)

Suck your abdomen inward and upward and exhale through your mouth.

When your abdomen is squeezed inward, close your mouth and continue exhaling through your nose.

While exhaling through the nose, do all the contractions:

Contract your anterior and posterior openings.

Squeeze the ball with your knees.

Squeeze the balls with your fingers.

Press your tongue to your palate (close your mouth and clench your teeth).

Contract your nostrils.

Your eyes look upward, open (don't contract your forehead; feel as if all the muscles are pulling upward in the direction of your eyes).

Relaxation (inhaling)

Inhale slowly through your nose, fill your lungs with air right into the abdominal cavity, and relax all the contractions.

The movements flow harmoniously.

Repetition

Repeat the relaxation and contraction using the slow technique about 10 times.

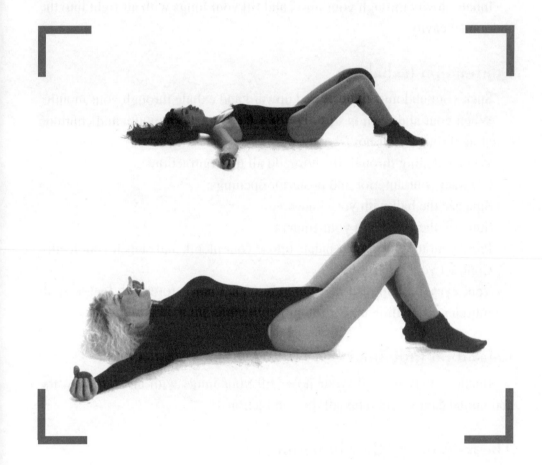

Exercise number 3:

Lie on your back, legs bent, arms stretched behind your head, knees holding a ball, and each hand holding a ball. (See picture.)

Relaxation (inhaling)

Inhale slowly through your nose, and fill your lungs with air right into the abdominal cavity.

Contraction (exhaling)

Suck your abdomen inward and upward and exhale through your mouth.

When your abdomen is squeezed inward, close your mouth and continue exhaling through your nose.

While exhaling through the nose, do all the contractions:

Contract your anterior and posterior openings.

Squeeze the ball with your knees.

Squeeze the balls with your fingers.

Press your tongue to your palate (close your mouth and clench your teeth).

Contract your nostrils.

Your eyes look upward, open (don't contract your forehead; feel as if all the muscles are pulling upward in the direction of your eyes).

Relaxation (inhaling)

Inhale slowly through your nose, fill your lungs with air right into the abdominal cavity, and relax all the contractions.

The movements flow harmoniously.

Repetition

Repeat the relaxation and contraction using the slow technique about 10 times.

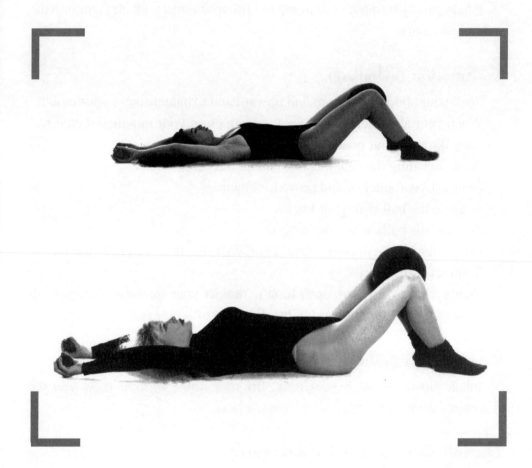

Exercise number 4:

Lie on your back, legs straight, arms at the sides of your body, knees holding a ball, and each hand holding a ball. (See picture.)

Relaxation (inhaling)

Inhale slowly through your nose, and fill your lungs with air right into the abdominal cavity.

Contraction (exhaling)

Suck your abdomen inward and upward and exhale through your mouth.

When your abdomen is squeezed inward, close your mouth and continue exhaling through your nose.

While exhaling through the nose, do all the contractions:

Contract your anterior and posterior openings.

Squeeze the ball with your knees.

Squeeze the balls with your fingers.

Press your tongue to your palate (close your mouth and clench your teeth).

Contract your nostrils.

Your eyes look upward, open (don't contract your forehead; feel as if all the muscles are pulling upward in the direction of your eyes).

Relaxation (inhaling)

Inhale slowly through your nose, fill your lungs with air right into the abdominal cavity, and relax all the contractions.

The movements flow harmoniously.

Repetition

Repeat the relaxation and contraction using the slow technique about 10 times.

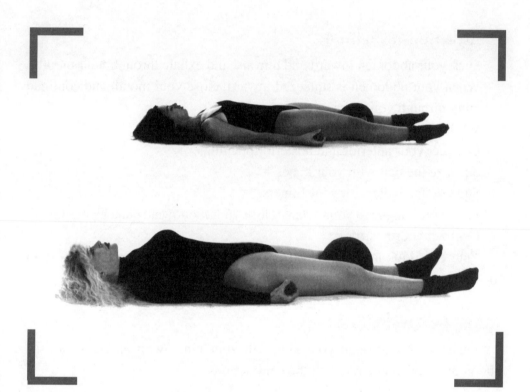

Exercise number 5:

Lie on your back, legs straight, arms straight out, knees holding a ball, and each hand holding a ball. (See picture.)

Relaxation (inhaling)

Inhale slowly through your nose, and fill your lungs with air right into the abdominal cavity.

Contraction (exhaling)

Suck your abdomen inward and upward and exhale through your mouth.

When your abdomen is squeezed inward, close your mouth and continue exhaling through your nose.

While exhaling through the nose, do all the contractions:

Contract your anterior and posterior openings.

Squeeze the ball with your knees.

Squeeze the balls with your fingers.

Press your tongue to your palate (close your mouth and clench your teeth).

Contract your nostrils.

Your eyes look upward, open (don't contract your forehead; feel as if all the muscles are pulling upward in the direction of your eyes).

Relaxation (inhaling)

Inhale slowly through your nose, fill your lungs with air right into the abdominal cavity, and relax all the contractions.

The movements flow harmoniously.

Repetition

Repeat the relaxation and contraction using the slow technique about 10 times.

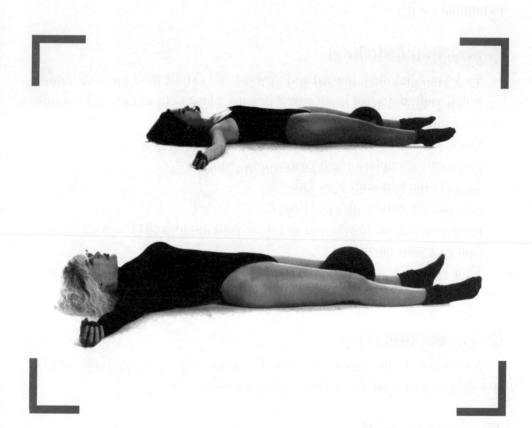

Exercise number 6:

Lie on your back, legs straight, arms stretched behind your head, knees holding a ball, and each hand holding a ball. (See picture.)

Relaxation (inhaling)

Inhale slowly through your nose, and fill your lungs with air right into the abdominal cavity.

Contraction (exhaling)

Suck your abdomen inward and upward and exhale through your mouth.

When your abdomen is squeezed inward, close your mouth and continue exhaling through your nose.

While exhaling through the nose, do all the contractions:

Contract your anterior and posterior openings.

Squeeze the ball with your knees.

Squeeze the balls with your fingers.

Press your tongue to your palate (close your mouth and clench your teeth).

Contract your nostrils.

Your eyes look upward, open (don't contract your forehead; feel as if all the muscles are pulling upward in the direction of your eyes).

Relaxation (inhaling)

Inhale slowly through your nose, fill your lungs with air right into the abdominal cavity, and relax all the contractions.

The movements flow harmoniously.

Repetition

Repeat the relaxation and contraction using the slow technique about 10 times.

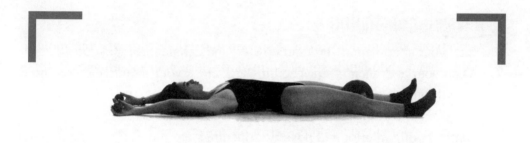

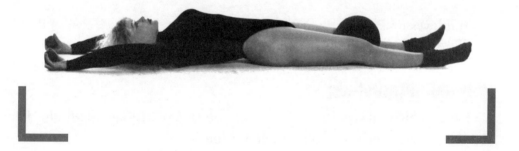

Exercise number 7:

Lie on your back, legs straight, arms at the sides of your body, feet holding a ball, and each hand holding a ball. (See picture.)

Relaxation (inhaling)

Inhale slowly through your nose, and fill your lungs with air right into the abdominal cavity.

Contraction (exhaling)

Suck your abdomen inward and upward and exhale through your mouth.

When your abdomen is squeezed inward, close your mouth and continue exhaling through your nose.

While exhaling through the nose, do all the contractions:

Contract your anterior and posterior openings.

Squeeze the ball with your feet.

Squeeze the balls with your fingers.

Press your tongue to your palate (close your mouth and clench your teeth).

Contract your nostrils.

Your eyes look upward, open (don't contract your forehead; feel as if all the muscles are pulling upward in the direction of your eyes).

Relaxation (inhaling)

Inhale slowly through your nose, fill your lungs with air right into the abdominal cavity, and relax all the contractions.

The movements flow harmoniously.

Repetition

Repeat the relaxation and contraction using the slow technique about 10 times.

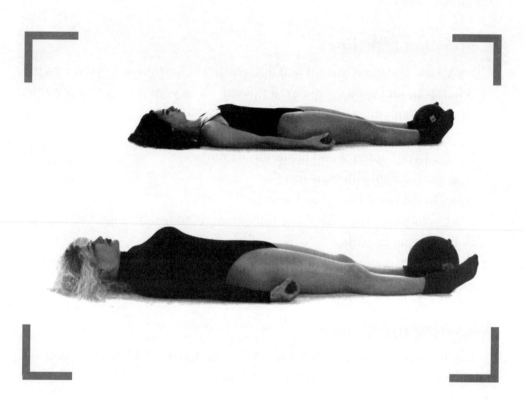

Exercise number 8:

Lie on your back, legs straight, arms straight out, feet holding a ball, and each hand holding a ball. (See picture.)

Relaxation (inhaling)

Inhale slowly through your nose, and fill your lungs with air right into the abdominal cavity.

Contraction (exhaling)

Suck your abdomen inward and upward and exhale through your mouth.

When your abdomen is squeezed inward, close your mouth and continue exhaling through your nose.

While exhaling through the nose, do all the contractions:

Contract your anterior and posterior openings.

Squeeze the ball with your feet.

Squeeze the balls with your fingers.

Press your tongue to your palate (close your mouth and clench your teeth).

Contract your nostrils.

Your eyes look upward, open (don't contract your forehead; feel as if all the muscles are pulling upward in the direction of your eyes).

Relaxation (inhaling)

Inhale slowly through your nose, fill your lungs with air right into the abdominal cavity, and relax all the contractions.

The movements flow harmoniously.

Repetition

Repeat the relaxation and contraction using the slow technique about 10 times.

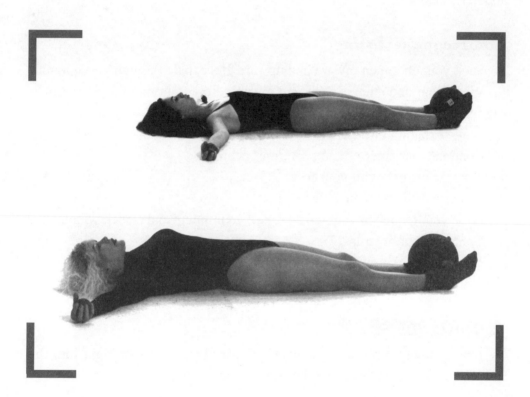

Exercise number 9:

Lie on your back, legs straight, arms stretched behind your head, feet holding a ball, and each hand holding a ball. (See picture.)

Relaxation (inhaling)

Inhale slowly through your nose, and fill your lungs with air right into the abdominal cavity.

Contraction (exhaling)

Suck your abdomen inward and upward and exhale through your mouth.

When your abdomen is squeezed inward, close your mouth and continue exhaling through your nose.

While exhaling through the nose, do all the contractions:

Contract your anterior and posterior openings.

Squeeze the ball with your feet.

Squeeze the balls with your fingers.

Press your tongue to your palate (close your mouth and clench your teeth).

Contract your nostrils.

Your eyes look upward, open (don't contract your forehead; feel as if all the muscles are pulling upward in the direction of your eyes).

Relaxation (inhaling)

Inhale slowly through your nose, fill your lungs with air right into the abdominal cavity, and relax all the contractions.

The movements flow harmoniously.

Repetition

Repeat the relaxation and contraction using the slow technique about 10 times.

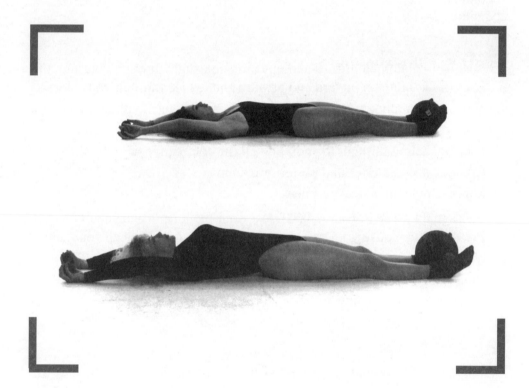

Exercise number 10:

Lie on your back, legs straight up at a 90-degree angle, arms at the sides of your body, knees holding a ball, and each hand holding a ball. (See picture.)

Relaxation (inhaling)

Inhale slowly through your nose, and fill your lungs with air right into the abdominal cavity.

Contraction (exhaling)

Suck your abdomen inward and upward and exhale through your mouth.

When your abdomen is squeezed inward, close your mouth and continue exhaling through your nose.

While exhaling through the nose, do all the contractions:

Contract your anterior and posterior openings.

Squeeze the ball with your knees.

Squeeze the balls with your fingers.

Press your tongue to your palate (close your mouth and clench your teeth).

Contract your nostrils.

Your eyes look upward, open (don't contract your forehead; feel as if all the muscles are pulling upward in the direction of your eyes).

Relaxation (inhaling)

Inhale slowly through your nose, fill your lungs with air right into the abdominal cavity, and relax all the contractions.

The movements flow harmoniously.

Repetition

Repeat the relaxation and contraction using the slow technique about 10 times.

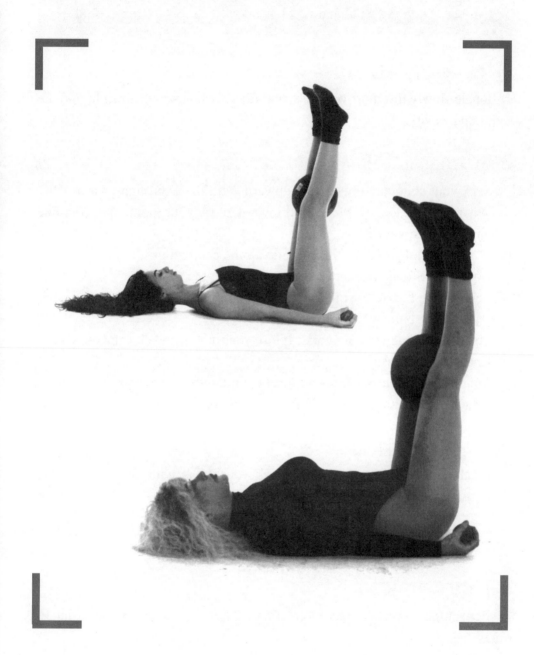

Exercise number 11:

Lie on your back, legs straight up at a 90-degree angle, arms straight out, knees holding a ball, and each hand holding a ball. (See picture.)

Relaxation (inhaling)

Inhale slowly through your nose, and fill your lungs with air right into the abdominal cavity.

Contraction (exhaling)

Suck your abdomen inward and upward and exhale through your mouth.

When your abdomen is squeezed inward, close your mouth and continue exhaling through your nose.

While exhaling through the nose, do all the contractions:

Contract your anterior and posterior openings.

Squeeze the ball with your knees.

Squeeze the balls with your fingers.

Press your tongue to your palate (close your mouth and clench your teeth).

Contract your nostrils.

Your eyes look upward, open (don't contract your forehead; feel as if all the muscles are pulling upward in the direction of your eyes).

Relaxation (inhaling)

Inhale slowly through your nose, fill your lungs with air right into the abdominal cavity, and relax all the contractions.

The movements flow harmoniously.

Repetition

Repeat the relaxation and contraction using the slow technique about 10 times.

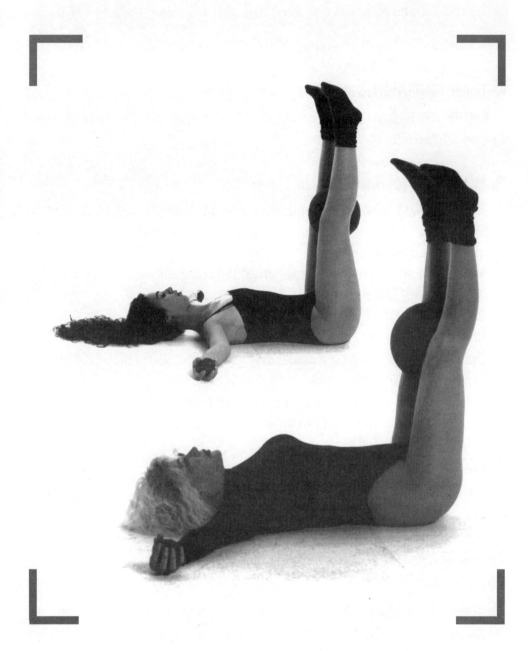

Exercise number 12:

Lie on your back, legs straight up at a 90-degree angle, arms stretched behind your head, knees holding a ball, and each hand holding a ball. (See picture.)

Relaxation (inhaling)

Inhale slowly through your nose, and fill your lungs with air right into the abdominal cavity.

Contraction (exhaling)

Suck your abdomen inward and upward and exhale through your mouth.

When your abdomen is squeezed inward, close your mouth and continue exhaling through your nose.

While exhaling through the nose, do all the contractions:

Contract your anterior and posterior openings.

Squeeze the ball with your knees.

Squeeze the balls with your fingers.

Press your tongue to your palate (close your mouth and clench your teeth).

Contract your nostrils.

Your eyes look upward, open (don't contract your forehead; feel as if all the muscles are pulling upward in the direction of your eyes).

Relaxation (inhaling)

Inhale slowly through your nose, fill your lungs with air right into the abdominal cavity, and relax all the contractions.

The movements flow harmoniously.

Repetition

Repeat the relaxation and contraction using the slow technique about 10 times.

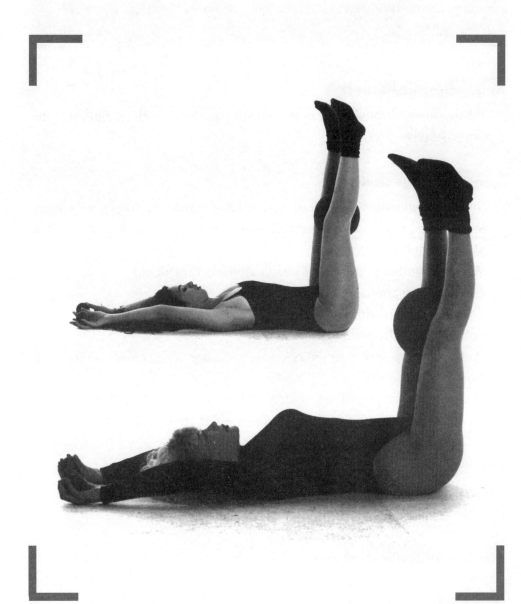

Exercise number 13:

Lie on your back, legs straight up at a 90-degree angle, arms at the sides of your body, feet holding a ball, and each hand holding a ball. (See picture.)

Relaxation (inhaling)

Inhale slowly through your nose, and fill your lungs with air right into the abdominal cavity.

Contraction (exhaling)

Suck your abdomen inward and upward and exhale through your mouth.

When your abdomen is squeezed inward, close your mouth and continue exhaling through your nose.

While exhaling through the nose, do all the contractions:

Contract your anterior and posterior openings.

Squeeze the ball with your feet.

Squeeze the balls with your fingers.

Press your tongue to your palate (close your mouth and clench your teeth).

Contract your nostrils.

Your eyes look upward, open (don't contract your forehead; feel as if all the muscles are pulling upward in the direction of your eyes).

Relaxation (inhaling)

Inhale slowly through your nose, fill your lungs with air right into the abdominal cavity, and relax all the contractions.

The movements flow harmoniously.

Repetition

Repeat the relaxation and contraction using the slow technique about 10 times.

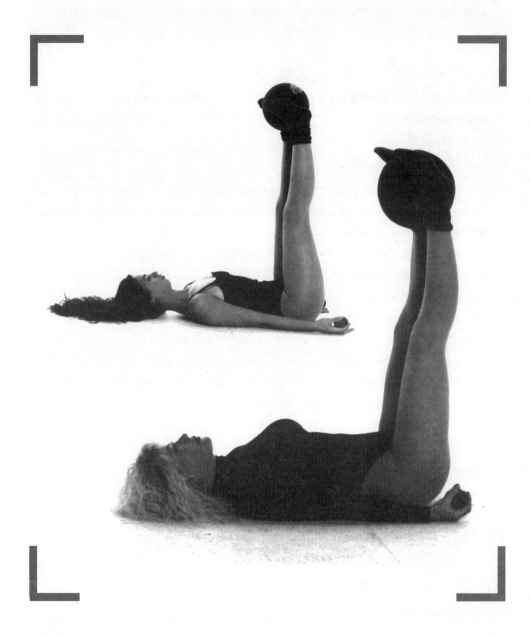

Exercise number 14:

Lie on your back, legs straight up at a 90-degree angle, arms straight out, feet holding a ball, and each hand holding a ball. (See picture.)

Relaxation (inhaling)

Inhale slowly through your nose, and fill your lungs with air right into the abdominal cavity.

Contraction (exhaling)

Suck your abdomen inward and upward and exhale through your mouth.

When your abdomen is squeezed inward, close your mouth and continue exhaling through your nose.

While exhaling through the nose, do all the contractions:

Contract your anterior and posterior openings.

Squeeze the ball with your feet.

Squeeze the balls with your fingers.

Press your tongue to your palate (close your mouth and clench your teeth).

Contract your nostrils.

Your eyes look upward, open (don't contract your forehead; feel as if all the muscles are pulling upward in the direction of your eyes).

Relaxation (inhaling)

Inhale slowly through your nose, fill your lungs with air right into the abdominal cavity, and relax all the contractions.

The movements flow harmoniously.

Repetition

Repeat the relaxation and contraction using the slow technique about 10 times.

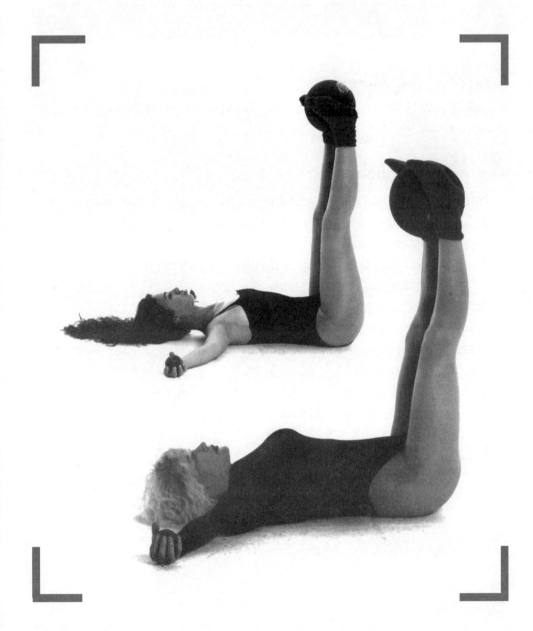

Exercise number 15:

Lie on your back, legs straight up at a 90-degree angle, arms stretched behind your head, feet holding a ball, and each hand holding a ball. (See picture.)

Relaxation (inhaling)

Inhale slowly through your nose, and fill your lungs with air right into the abdominal cavity.

Contraction (exhaling)

Suck your abdomen inward and upward and exhale through your mouth.

When your abdomen is squeezed inward, close your mouth and continue exhaling through your nose.

While exhaling through the nose, do all the contractions:

Contract your anterior and posterior openings.

Squeeze the ball with your feet.

Squeeze the balls with your fingers.

Press your tongue to your palate (close your mouth and clench your teeth).

Contract your nostrils.

Your eyes look upward, open (don't contract your forehead; feel as if all the muscles are pulling upward in the direction of your eyes).

Relaxation (inhaling)

Inhale slowly through your nose, fill your lungs with air right into the abdominal cavity, and relax all the contractions.

The movements flow harmoniously.

Repetition

Repeat the relaxation and contraction using the slow technique about 10 times.

N.B.

It is important and advisable to perform the exercise program, 1-15, for the first day of the second week, every day.

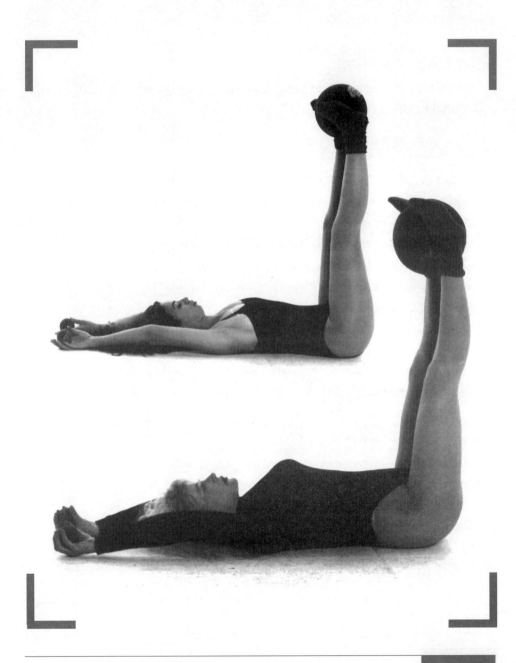

Second week: second day

Exercise number 1:

Lie on your back, legs bent, arms stretched upward holding a ball, and knees holding a ball. (See picture.)

Relaxation (inhaling)

Inhale slowly through your nose, and fill your lungs with air right into the abdominal cavity.

Contraction (exhaling)

Suck your abdomen inward and upward and exhale through your mouth.

When your abdomen is squeezed inward, close your mouth and continue exhaling through your nose.

While exhaling through the nose, do all the contractions:

Contract your anterior and posterior openings.

Squeeze the ball with your knees.

Squeeze the ball with your hands.

Press your tongue to your palate (close your mouth and clench your teeth).

Contract your nostrils.

Your eyes look upward, open (don't contract your forehead; feel as if all the muscles are pulling upward in the direction of your eyes).

Relaxation (inhaling)

Inhale slowly through your nose, fill your lungs with air right into the abdominal cavity, and relax all the contractions.

The movements flow harmoniously.

Repetition

Repeat the relaxation and contraction using the slow technique about 10 times.

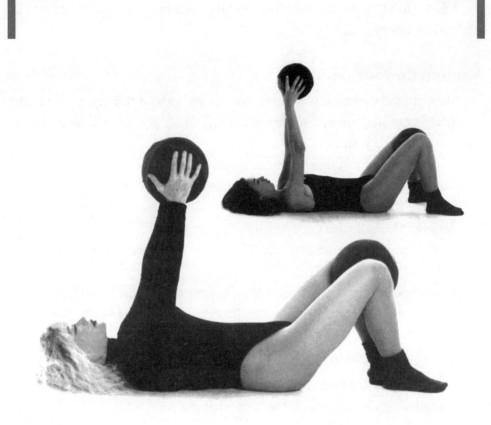

Exercise number 2:

Lie on your back, legs bent, arms stretched behind your head, holding a ball, and knees holding a ball. (See picture.)

Relaxation (inhaling)

Inhale slowly through your nose, and fill your lungs with air right into the abdominal cavity.

Contraction (exhaling)

Suck your abdomen inward and upward and exhale through your mouth.

When your abdomen is squeezed inward, close your mouth and continue exhaling through your nose.

While exhaling through the nose, do all the contractions:

Contract your anterior and posterior openings.

Squeeze the ball with your knees.

Squeeze the ball with your hands.

Press your tongue to your palate (close your mouth and clench your teeth).

Contract your nostrils.

Your eyes look upward, open (don't contract your forehead; feel as if all the muscles are pulling upward in the direction of your eyes).

Relaxation (inhaling)

Inhale slowly through your nose, fill your lungs with air right into the abdominal cavity, and relax all the contractions.

The movements flow harmoniously.

Repetition

Repeat the relaxation and contraction using the slow technique about 10 times.

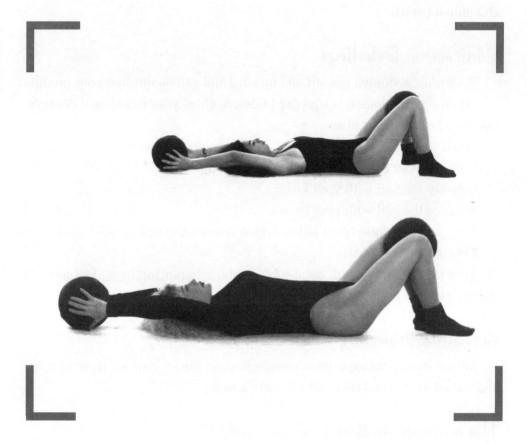

Exercise number 3:

Lie on your back, legs straight, arms straight up holding a ball, and knees holding a ball. (See picture.)

Relaxation (inhaling)

Inhale slowly through your nose, and fill your lungs with air right into the abdominal cavity.

Contraction (exhaling)

Suck your abdomen inward and upward and exhale through your mouth.

When your abdomen is squeezed inward, close your mouth and continue exhaling through your nose.

While exhaling through the nose, do all the contractions:

Contract your anterior and posterior openings.

Squeeze the ball with your knees.

Squeeze the ball with your hands.

Press your tongue to your palate (close your mouth and clench your teeth).

Contract your nostrils.

Your eyes look upward, open (don't contract your forehead; feel as if all the muscles are pulling upward in the direction of your eyes).

Relaxation (inhaling)

Inhale slowly through your nose, fill your lungs with air right into the abdominal cavity, and relax all the contractions.

The movements flow harmoniously.

Repetition

Repeat the relaxation and contraction using the slow technique about 10 times.

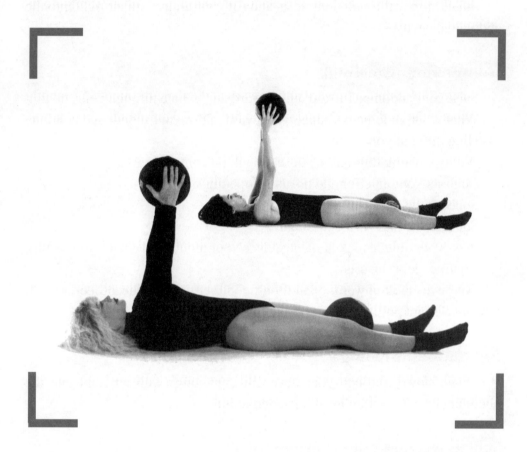

Exercise number 4:

Lie on your back, legs straight, arms stretched behind the head, holding a ball, and knees holding a ball. (See picture.)

Relaxation (inhaling)

Inhale slowly through your nose, and fill your lungs with air right into the abdominal cavity.

Contraction (exhaling)

Suck your abdomen inward and upward and exhale through your mouth.

When your abdomen is squeezed inward, close your mouth and continue exhaling through your nose.

While exhaling through the nose, do all the contractions:

Contract your anterior and posterior openings.

Squeeze the ball with your knees.

Squeeze the ball with your hands.

Press your tongue to your palate (close your mouth and clench your teeth).

Contract your nostrils.

Your eyes look upward, open (don't contract your forehead; feel as if all the muscles are pulling upward in the direction of your eyes).

Relaxation (inhaling)

Inhale slowly through your nose, fill your lungs with air right into the abdominal cavity, and relax all the contractions.

The movements flow harmoniously.

Repetition

Repeat the relaxation and contraction using the slow technique about 10 times.

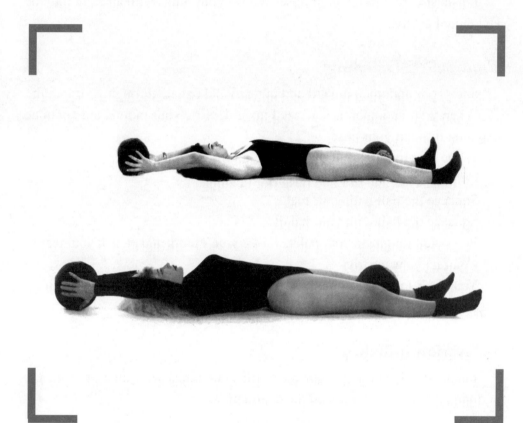

Exercise number 5:

Lie on your back, legs straight, arms straight up holding a ball, and feet holding a ball. (See picture.)

Relaxation (inhaling)

Inhale slowly through your nose, and fill your lungs with air right into the abdominal cavity.

Contraction (exhaling)

Suck your abdomen inward and upward and exhale through your mouth.

When your abdomen is squeezed inward, close your mouth and continue exhaling through your nose.

While exhaling through the nose, do all the contractions:

Contract your anterior and posterior openings.

Squeeze the ball with your feet.

Squeeze the ball with your hands.

Press your tongue to your palate (close your mouth and clench your teeth).

Contract your nostrils.

Your eyes look upward, open (don't contract your forehead; feel as if all the muscles are pulling upward in the direction of your eyes).

Relaxation (inhaling)

Inhale slowly through your nose, fill your lungs with air right into the abdominal cavity, and relax all the contractions.

The movements flow harmoniously.

Repetition

Repeat the relaxation and contraction using the slow technique about 10 times.

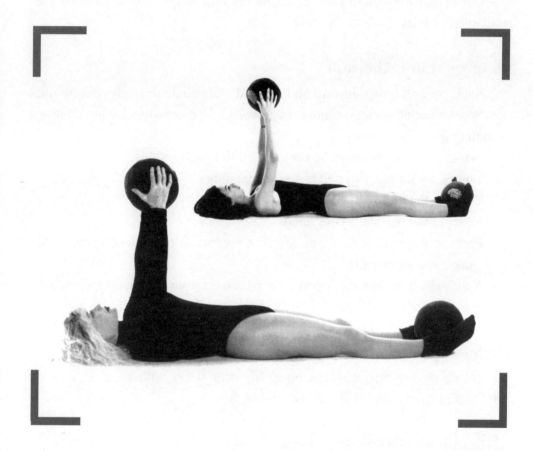

Exercise number 6:

Lie on your back, legs straight, arms stretched behind your head, holding a ball, and feet holding a ball. (See picture.)

Relaxation (inhaling)

Inhale slowly through your nose, and fill your lungs with air right into the abdominal cavity.

Contraction (exhaling)

Suck your abdomen inward and upward and exhale through your mouth.

When your abdomen is squeezed inward, close your mouth and continue exhaling through your nose.

While exhaling through the nose, do all the contractions:

Contract your anterior and posterior openings.

Squeeze the ball with your feet.

Squeeze the ball with your hands.

Press your tongue to your palate (close your mouth and clench your teeth).

Contract your nostrils.

Your eyes look upward, open (don't contract your forehead; feel as if all the muscles are pulling upward in the direction of your eyes).

Relaxation (inhaling)

Inhale slowly through your nose, fill your lungs with air right into the abdominal cavity, and relax all the contractions.

The movements flow harmoniously.

Repetition

Repeat the relaxation and contraction using the slow technique about 10 times.

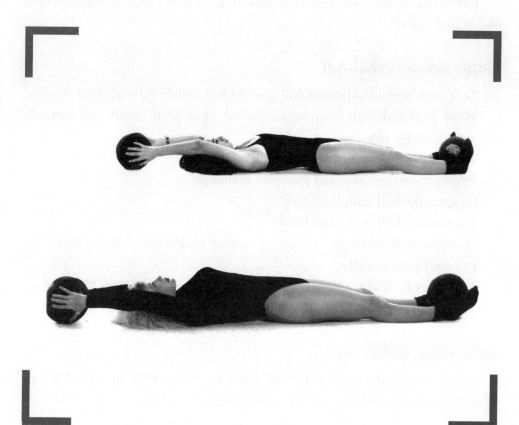

Exercise number 7:

Lie on your back, legs straight up at a 90-degree angle, arms straight up holding a ball, and knees holding a ball. (See picture.)

Relaxation (inhaling)

Inhale slowly through your nose, and fill your lungs with air right into the abdominal cavity.

Contraction (exhaling)

Suck your abdomen inward and upward and exhale through your mouth.

When your abdomen is squeezed inward, close your mouth and continue exhaling through your nose.

While exhaling through the nose, do all the contractions:

Contract your anterior and posterior openings.

Squeeze the ball with your knees.

Squeeze the ball with your hands.

Press your tongue to your palate (close your mouth and clench your teeth).

Contract your nostrils.

Your eyes look upward, open (don't contract your forehead; feel as if all the muscles are pulling upward in the direction of your eyes).

Relaxation (inhaling)

Inhale slowly through your nose, fill your lungs with air right into the abdominal cavity, and relax all the contractions.

The movements flow harmoniously.

Repetition

Repeat the relaxation and contraction using the slow technique about 10 times.

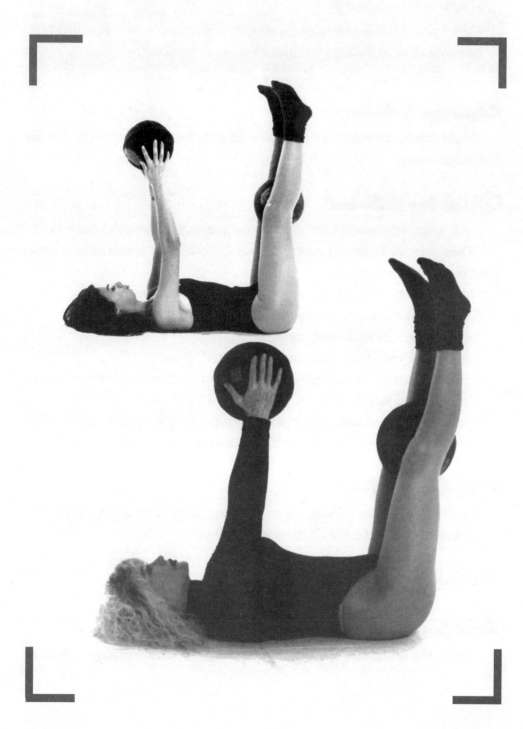

Exercise number 8:

Lie on your back, legs straight up at a 90-degree angle, arms stretched behind your head, holding a ball, and knees holding a ball. (See picture.)

Relaxation (inhaling)

Inhale slowly through your nose, and fill your lungs with air right into the abdominal cavity.

Contraction (exhaling)

Suck your abdomen inward and upward and exhale through your mouth.

When your abdomen is squeezed inward, close your mouth and continue exhaling through your nose.

While exhaling through the nose, do all the contractions:

Contract your anterior and posterior openings.

Squeeze the ball with your knees.

Squeeze the ball with your hands.

Press your tongue to your palate (close your mouth and clench your teeth).

Contract your nostrils.

Your eyes look upward, open (don't contract your forehead; feel as if all the muscles are pulling upward in the direction of your eyes).

Relaxation (inhaling)

Inhale slowly through your nose, fill your lungs with air right into the abdominal cavity, and relax all the contractions.

The movements flow harmoniously.

Repetition

Repeat the relaxation and contraction using the slow technique about 10 times.

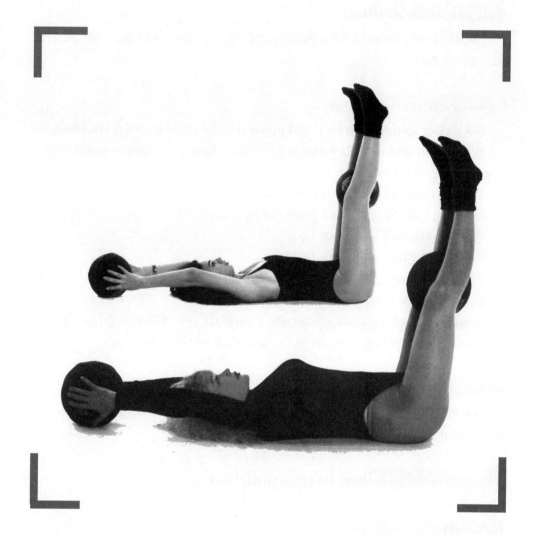

Exercise number 9:

Lie on your back, legs straight up at a 90-degree angle, arms straight up holding a ball, and feet holding a ball. (See picture.)

Relaxation (inhaling)

Inhale slowly through your nose, and fill your lungs with air right into the abdominal cavity.

Contraction (exhaling)

Suck your abdomen inward and upward and exhale through your mouth.

When your abdomen is squeezed inward, close your mouth and continue exhaling through your nose.

While exhaling through the nose, do all the contractions:

Contract your anterior and posterior openings.

Squeeze the ball with your feet.

Squeeze the ball with your hands.

Press your tongue to your palate (close your mouth and clench your teeth).

Contract your nostrils.

Your eyes look upward, open (don't contract your forehead; feel as if all the muscles are pulling upward in the direction of your eyes).

Relaxation (inhaling)

Inhale slowly through your nose, fill your lungs with air right into the abdominal cavity, and relax all the contractions.

The movements flow harmoniously.

Repetition

Repeat the relaxation and contraction using the slow technique about 10 times.

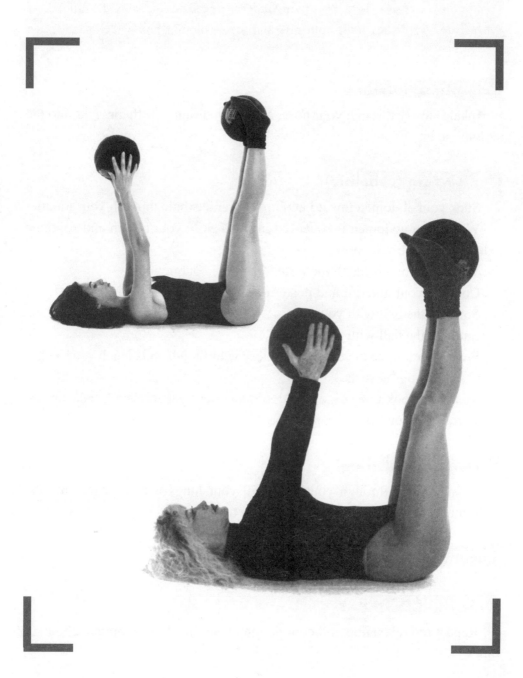

Exercise number 10:

Lie on your back, legs straight up at a 90-degree angle, arms stretched behind your head, holding a ball, and feet holding a ball. (See picture.)

Relaxation (inhaling)

Inhale slowly through your nose, and fill your lungs with air right into the abdominal cavity.

Contraction (exhaling)

Suck your abdomen inward and upward and exhale through your mouth.

When your abdomen is squeezed inward, close your mouth and continue exhaling through your nose.

While exhaling through the nose, do all the contractions:

Contract your anterior and posterior openings.

Squeeze the ball with your feet.

Squeeze the ball with your hands.

Press your tongue to your palate (close your mouth and clench your teeth).

Contract your nostrils.

Your eyes look upward, open (don't contract your forehead; feel as if all the muscles are pulling upward in the direction of your eyes).

Relaxation (inhaling)

Inhale slowly through your nose, fill your lungs with air right into the abdominal cavity, and relax all the contractions.

The movements flow harmoniously.

Repetition

Repeat the relaxation and contraction using the slow technique about 10 times.

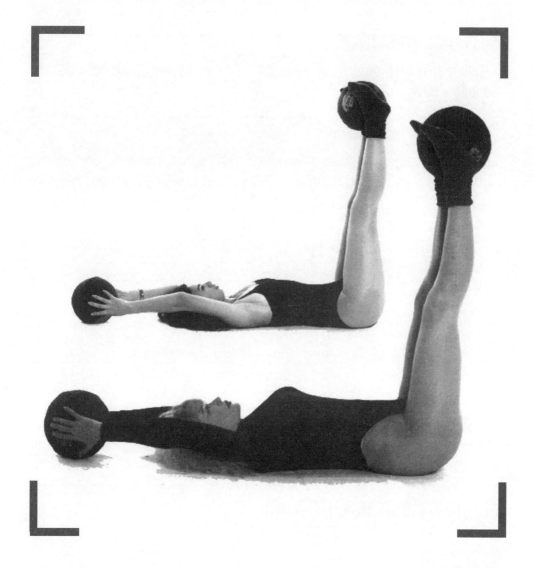

Now that you are familiar with this system of exercises, and you know how long it takes you, you can begin to create your own exercise schedule.

_____

_____

_____

_____

_____

_____

_____

_____

_____

_____

_____

_____

_____

_____

Exercises for Women

Second week: third day

Asymmetrical exercises:

Repeat all the exercises you have learned until now according to the order of the first and second days, once with the right side contracted and the left relaxed, and once with the left side contracted and the right relaxed.

Example

Third day: Exercise number 1:

Lie on your back, legs bent, arms at the side of your body, knees holding a ball, and each hand holding a ball.

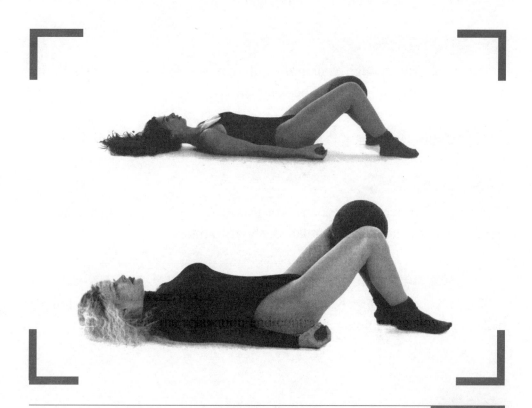

Relaxation (inhaling)

Inhale slowly through your nose, and fill your lungs with air right into the abdominal cavity.

Contraction (exhaling)

Suck your abdomen inward and upward and exhale through your mouth.

When your abdomen is squeezed inward, close your mouth and continue exhaling through your nose.

While exhaling through the nose, do all the contractions of the right side while the left side relaxes:

Contract your anterior and posterior openings on the right side / left side relaxed.

Squeeze the ball with your right knee / left knee relaxed.

Squeeze the ball with your right hand / left hand relaxed.

Press your tongue to your palate (close your mouth and clench your teeth).

Contract your right nostril / left side relaxed.

Your eyes look upward and to the right.

Relaxation (inhaling)

Inhale slowly through your nose, fill your lungs with air right into the abdominal cavity, and relax all the contractions.

The movements flow harmoniously.

Repetition

Repeat the relaxation and contraction using the slow asymmetrical technique right side contracted, left side relaxed, about 10 times.

Changing sides -- left side contracted and right side relaxed.

Lie on your back, legs bent, arms at the side of your body, knees holding a ball, and each hand holding a ball.

Relaxation (inhaling)

Inhale slowly through your nose, and fill your lungs with air right into the abdominal cavity.

Contraction (exhaling)

Suck your abdomen inward and upward and exhale through your mouth.

When your abdomen is squeezed inward, close your mouth and continue exhaling through your nose.

While exhaling through the nose, do all the contractions of the left side while the right side relaxes:

Contract your anterior and posterior openings on the left side / right side relaxed.

Squeeze the ball with your left knee / right knee relaxed.

Squeeze the ball with your left hand / right hand relaxed.

Press your tongue to your palate (close your mouth and clench your teeth).

Contract your left nostril / right side relaxed.

Your eyes look upward and to the left.

Relaxation (inhaling)

Inhale slowly through your nose, fill your lungs with air right into the abdominal cavity, and relax all the contractions.

The movements flow harmoniously.

Repetition

Repeat the relaxation and contraction using the slow asymmetrical technique, left side contracted, right side relaxed, about 10 times.

Repeat exercises 1-15 lying on your back using the slow technique 5 times, and the slow asymmetrical technique twice on each side - once on the right, and once on the left.

Second week: fourth day

Exercise number 1:

Lie on your right side, legs bent, knees holding a ball, right arm straight up above your head, holding a ball, head resting on the right arm, left arm straight along the side of your body, holding a ball. (See picture.)

Relaxation (inhaling)

Inhale slowly through your nose, and fill your lungs with air right into the abdominal cavity.

Contraction (exhaling)

Suck your abdomen inward and upward and exhale through your mouth.

When your abdomen is squeezed inward, close your mouth and continue exhaling through your nose.

While exhaling through the nose, do all the contractions:

Contract your anterior and posterior openings.

Squeeze the ball with your knees.

Squeeze the balls with your fingers.

Press your tongue to your palate (close your mouth and clench your teeth).

Contract your nostrils.

Your eyes look upward, open (don't contract your forehead; feel as if all the muscles are pulling upward in the direction of your eyes).

Relaxation (inhaling)

Inhale slowly through your nose, fill your lungs with air right into the abdominal cavity, and relax all the contractions.

The movements flow harmoniously.

Exercises for Women

Repetition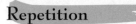

Repeat the relaxation and contraction using the slow technique about 10 times.

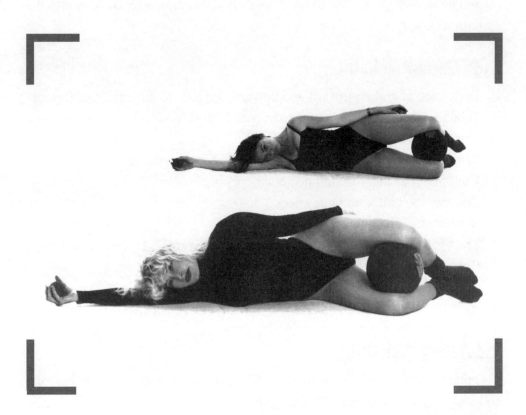

Exercise number 2:

Lie on your right side, legs straight, knees holding a ball, right arm straight up above your head, holding a ball, head resting on the right arm, left arm straight out in front of you, holding a ball. (See picture.)

Relaxation (inhaling)

Inhale slowly through your nose, and fill your lungs with air right into the abdominal cavity.

Contraction (exhaling)

Suck your abdomen inward and upward and exhale through your mouth.

When your abdomen is squeezed inward, close your mouth and continue exhaling through your nose.

While exhaling through the nose, do all the contractions:

Contract your anterior and posterior openings.

Squeeze the ball with your knees.

Squeeze the balls with your fingers.

Press your tongue to your palate (close your mouth and clench your teeth).

Contract your nostrils.

Your eyes look upward, open (don't contract your forehead; feel as if all the muscles are pulling upward in the direction of your eyes).

Relaxation (inhaling)

Inhale slowly through your nose, fill your lungs with air right into the abdominal cavity, and relax all the contractions.

The movements flow harmoniously.

Repetition

Repeat the relaxation and contraction using the slow technique about 10 times.

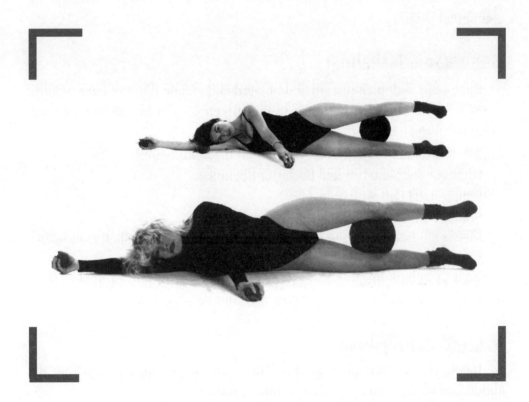

Exercise number 3:

Lie on your right side, legs straight, feet holding a ball, right arm straight up above your head, holding a ball, head resting on the right arm, left arm straight out in front of you, holding a ball. (See picture.)

Relaxation (inhaling)

Inhale slowly through your nose, and fill your lungs with air right into the abdominal cavity.

Contraction (exhaling)

Suck your abdomen inward and upward and exhale through your mouth.

When your abdomen is squeezed inward, close your mouth and continue exhaling through your nose.

While exhaling through the nose, do all the contractions:

Contract your anterior and posterior openings.

Squeeze the ball with your feet.

Squeeze the balls with your fingers.

Press your tongue to your palate (close your mouth and clench your teeth).

Contract your nostrils.

Your eyes look upward, open (don't contract your forehead; feel as if all the muscles are pulling upward in the direction of your eyes).

Relaxation (inhaling)

Inhale slowly through your nose, fill your lungs with air right into the abdominal cavity, and relax all the contractions.

The movements flow harmoniously.

Repetition

Repeat the relaxation and contraction using the slow technique about 10 times.

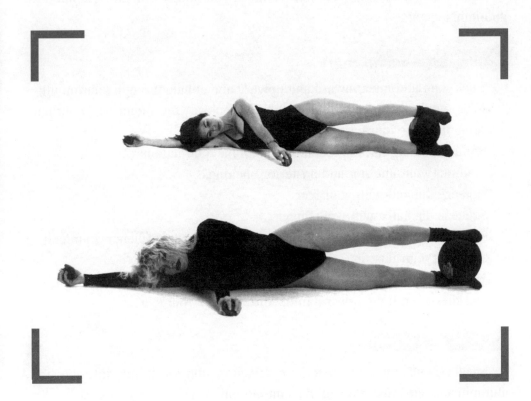

Exercise number 4:

Lie on your left side, legs bent, knees holding a ball, left arm straight up above your head, holding a ball, head resting on the left arm, right arm straight along the side of your body, holding a ball. (See picture.)

Relaxation (inhaling)

Inhale slowly through your nose, and fill your lungs with air right into the abdominal cavity.

Contraction (exhaling)

Suck your abdomen inward and upward and exhale through your mouth.

When your abdomen is squeezed inward, close your mouth and continue exhaling through your nose.

While exhaling through the nose, do all the contractions:

Contract your anterior and posterior openings.

Squeeze the ball with your knees.

Squeeze the balls with your fingers.

Press your tongue to your palate (close your mouth and clench your teeth).

Contract your nostrils.

Your eyes look upward, open (don't contract your forehead; feel as if all the muscles are pulling upward in the direction of your eyes).

Relaxation (inhaling)

Inhale slowly through your nose, fill your lungs with air right into the abdominal cavity, and relax all the contractions.

The movements flow harmoniously.

Repetition

Repeat the relaxation and contraction using the slow technique about 10 times.

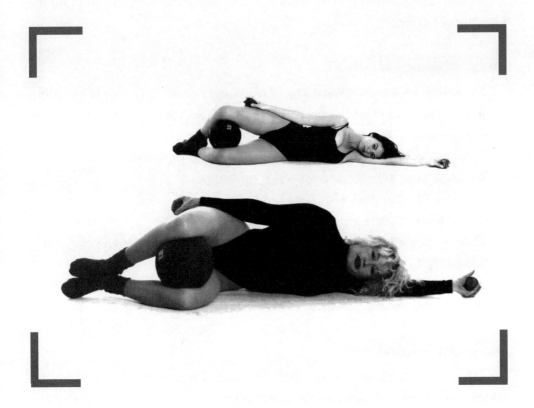

Exercise number 5:

Lie on your left side, legs straight, knees holding a ball, left arm straight up above your head, holding a ball, head resting on the left arm, right arm straight out in front of you, holding a ball. (See picture.)

Relaxation (inhaling)

Inhale slowly through your nose, and fill your lungs with air right into the abdominal cavity.

Contraction (exhaling)

Suck your abdomen inward and upward and exhale through your mouth.

When your abdomen is squeezed inward, close your mouth and continue exhaling through your nose.

While exhaling through the nose, do all the contractions:

Contract your anterior and posterior openings.

Squeeze the ball with your knees.

Squeeze the balls with your fingers.

Press your tongue to your palate (close your mouth and clench your teeth).

Contract your nostrils.

Your eyes look upward, open (don't contract your forehead; feel as if all the muscles are pulling upward in the direction of your eyes).

Relaxation (inhaling)

Inhale slowly through your nose, fill your lungs with air right into the abdominal cavity, and relax all the contractions.

The movements flow harmoniously.

Repetition

Repeat the relaxation and contraction using the slow technique about 10 times.

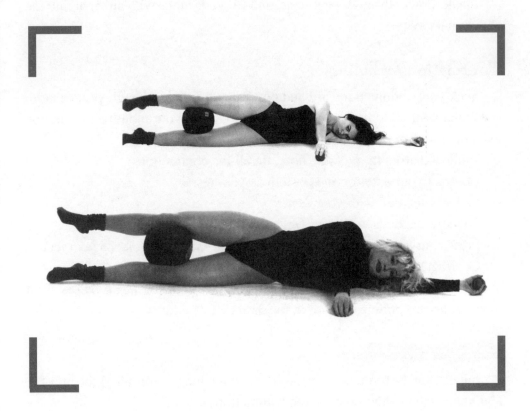

Exercise number 6:

Lie on your left side, legs straight, feet holding a ball, left arm straight up above your head, holding a ball, head resting on the left arm, right arm straight out in front of you, holding a ball. (See picture.)

Relaxation (inhaling)

Inhale slowly through your nose, and fill your lungs with air right into the abdominal cavity.

Contraction (exhaling)

Suck your abdomen inward and upward and exhale through your mouth.

When your abdomen is squeezed inward, close your mouth and continue exhaling through your nose.

While exhaling through the nose, do all the contractions:

Contract your anterior and posterior openings.

Squeeze the ball with your feet.

Squeeze the balls with your fingers.

Press your tongue to your palate (close your mouth and clench your teeth).

Contract your nostrils.

Your eyes look upward, open (don't contract your forehead; feel as if all the muscles are pulling upward in the direction of your eyes).

Relaxation (inhaling)

Inhale slowly through your nose, fill your lungs with air right into the abdominal cavity, and relax all the contractions.

The movements flow harmoniously.

Repetition

Repeat the relaxation and contraction using the slow technique about 10 times.

Repeat exercises 1-15 lying on your back, using the slow technique, five times.

Repeat the same exercises, using the slow asymmetrical technique twice - once on the right side, and once on the left.

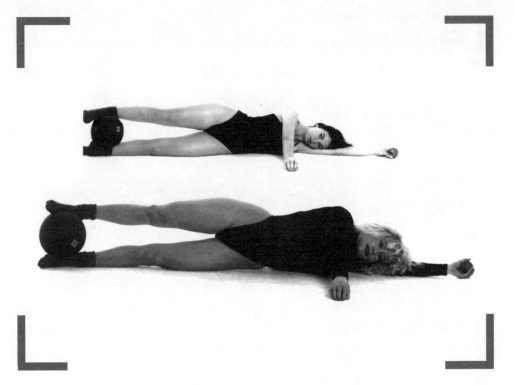

Second week: fifth day

Exercise number 1:

Lie on your stomach, legs bent, knees holding a ball, body supported by your elbows, each hand holding a ball. (See picture.)

Relaxation (inhaling)

Inhale slowly through your nose, and fill your lungs with air right into the abdominal cavity.

Contraction (exhaling)

Suck your abdomen inward and upward and exhale through your mouth.

When your abdomen is squeezed inward, close your mouth and continue exhaling through your nose.

While exhaling through the nose, do all the contractions:

Contract your anterior and posterior openings.

Squeeze the ball with your knees.

Squeeze the balls with your fingers.

Press your tongue to your palate (close your mouth and clench your teeth).

Contract your nostrils.

Your eyes look upward, open (don't contract your forehead; feel as if all the muscles are pulling upward in the direction of your eyes).

Relaxation (inhaling)

Inhale slowly through your nose, fill your lungs with air right into the abdominal cavity, and relax all the contractions.

The movements flow harmoniously.

Repetition

Repeat the relaxation and contraction using the slow technique about 10 times.

Exercises for Women

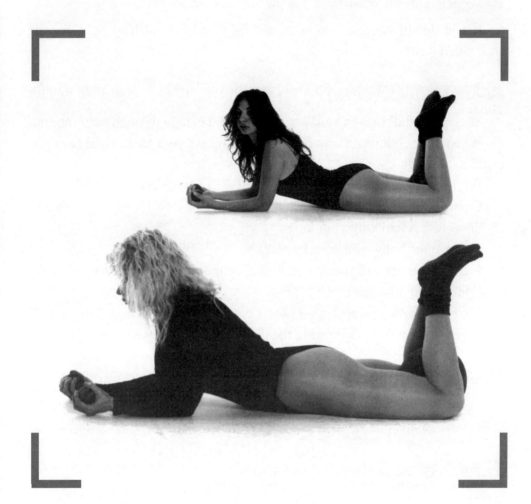

Exercise number 2:

Lie on your stomach, legs straight, knees holding a ball, body supported by your elbows, each hand holding a ball. (See picture.)

Relaxation (inhaling)

Inhale slowly through your nose, and fill your lungs with air right into the abdominal cavity.

Contraction (exhaling)

Suck your abdomen inward and upward and exhale through your mouth.

When your abdomen is squeezed inward, close your mouth and continue exhaling through your nose.

While exhaling through the nose, do all the contractions:

Contract your anterior and posterior openings.

Squeeze the ball with your knees.

Squeeze the balls with your fingers.

Press your tongue to your palate (close your mouth and clench your teeth).

Contract your nostrils.

Your eyes look upward, open (don't contract your forehead; feel as if all the muscles are pulling upward in the direction of your eyes).

Relaxation (inhaling)

Inhale slowly through your nose, fill your lungs with air right into the abdominal cavity, and relax all the contractions.

The movements flow harmoniously.

Repetition

Repeat the relaxation and contraction using the slow technique about 10 times.

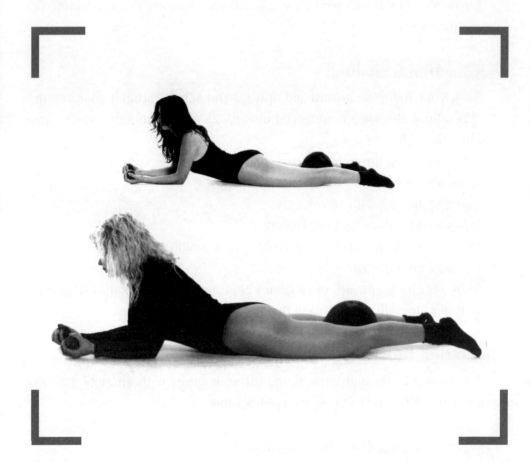

Exercise number 3:

Lie on your stomach, legs straight, feet holding a ball, body supported by your elbows, each hand holding a ball. (See picture.)

Relaxation (inhaling)

Inhale slowly through your nose, and fill your lungs with air right into the abdominal cavity.

Contraction (exhaling)

Suck your abdomen inward and upward and exhale through your mouth.

When your abdomen is squeezed inward, close your mouth and continue exhaling through your nose.

While exhaling through the nose, do all the contractions:

Contract your anterior and posterior openings.

Squeeze the ball with your feet.

Squeeze the balls with your fingers.

Press your tongue to your palate (close your mouth and clench your teeth).

Contract your nostrils.

Your eyes look upward, open (don't contract your forehead; feel as if all the muscles are pulling upward in the direction of your eyes).

Relaxation (inhaling)

Inhale slowly through your nose, fill your lungs with air right into the abdominal cavity, and relax all the contractions.

The movements flow harmoniously.

Repetition

Repeat the relaxation and contraction using the slow technique about 10 times.

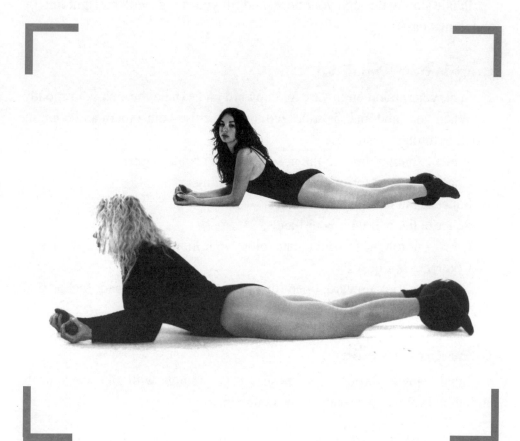

Exercise number 4:

Lie on your stomach, legs bent, knees holding a ball, arms stretched up above your head, holding a ball. (See picture.)

Relaxation (inhaling)

Inhale slowly through your nose, and fill your lungs with air right into the abdominal cavity.

Contraction (exhaling)

Suck your abdomen inward and upward and exhale through your mouth.

When your abdomen is squeezed inward, close your mouth and continue exhaling through your nose.

While exhaling through the nose, do all the contractions:

Contract your anterior and posterior openings.

Squeeze the ball with your knees.

Squeeze the ball with your hands.

Press your tongue to your palate (close your mouth and clench your teeth).

Contract your nostrils.

Your eyes look upward, open (don't contract your forehead; feel as if all the muscles are pulling upward in the direction of your eyes).

Relaxation (inhaling)

Inhale slowly through your nose, fill your lungs with air right into the abdominal cavity, and relax all the contractions.

The movements flow harmoniously.

Repetition

Repeat the relaxation and contraction using the slow technique about 10 times.

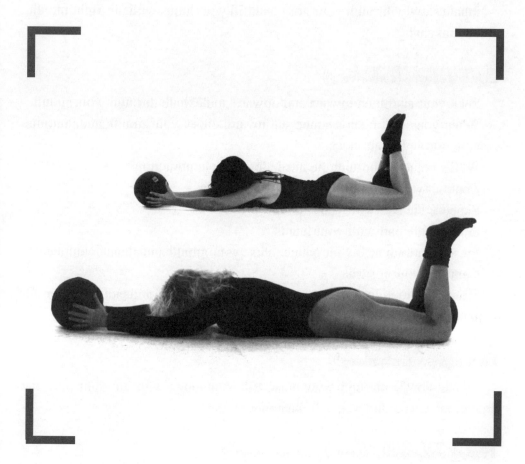

Exercise number 5:

Lie on your stomach, legs stretched out, knees holding a ball, arms stretched up above your head, holding a ball. (See picture.)

Relaxation (inhaling)

Inhale slowly through your nose, and fill your lungs with air right into the abdominal cavity.

Contraction (exhaling)

Suck your abdomen inward and upward and exhale through your mouth.

When your abdomen is squeezed inward, close your mouth and continue exhaling through your nose.

While exhaling through the nose, do all the contractions:

Contract your anterior and posterior openings.

Squeeze the ball with your knees.

Squeeze the ball with your hands.

Press your tongue to your palate (close your mouth and clench your teeth).

Contract your nostrils.

Your eyes look upward, open (don't contract your forehead; feel as if all the muscles are pulling upward in the direction of your eyes).

Relaxation (inhaling)

Inhale slowly through your nose, fill your lungs with air right into the abdominal cavity, and relax all the contractions.

The movements flow harmoniously.

Repetition

Repeat the relaxation and contraction using the slow technique about 10 times.

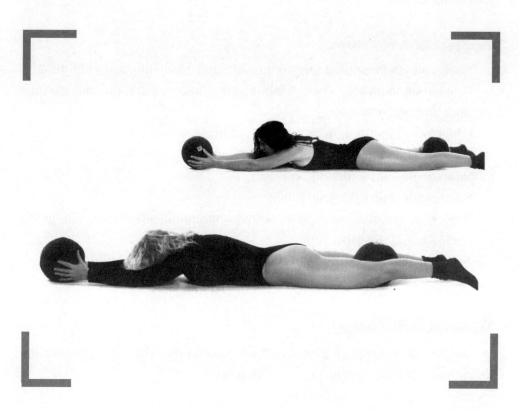

Exercise number 6:

Lie on your stomach, legs stretched out, feet holding a ball, arms stretched up above your head, holding a ball. (See picture.)

Relaxation (inhaling)

Inhale slowly through your nose, and fill your lungs with air right into the abdominal cavity.

Contraction (exhaling)

Suck your abdomen inward and upward and exhale through your mouth.

When your abdomen is squeezed inward, close your mouth and continue exhaling through your nose.

While exhaling through the nose, do all the contractions:

Contract your anterior and posterior openings.

Squeeze the ball with your feet.

Squeeze the ball with your hands.

Press your tongue to your palate (close your mouth and clench your teeth).

Contract your nostrils.

Your eyes look upward, open (don't contract your forehead; feel as if all the muscles are pulling upward in the direction of your eyes).

Relaxation (inhaling)

Inhale slowly through your nose, fill your lungs with air right into the abdominal cavity, and relax all the contractions.

The movements flow harmoniously.

Repetition

Repeat the relaxation and contraction using the slow technique about 10 times.

Repeat exercises 1-15 lying on your back, using the slow technique, five times.
Repeat the same exercises using the slow asymmetrical technique twice - once on the right side, and once on the left.

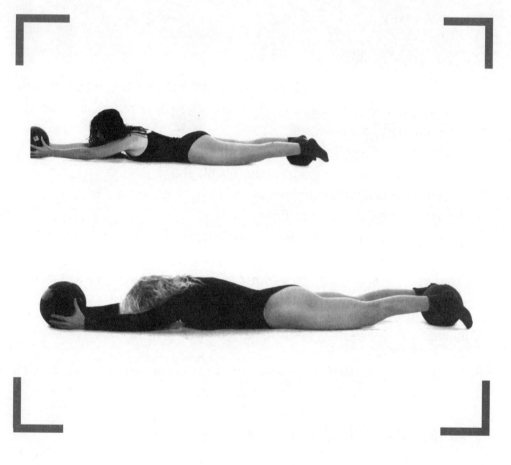

Second week: sixth day

Exercise number 1 - performed sitting on a chair:
Sit upright on a chair, feet on a footrest, knees holding a ball, arms straight down at your sides, each hand holding a ball. (See picture.)

Relaxation (inhaling)

Inhale slowly through your nose, and fill your lungs with air right into the abdominal cavity.

Contraction (exhaling)

Suck your abdomen inward and upward and exhale through your mouth.

When your abdomen is squeezed inward, close your mouth and continue exhaling through your nose.

While exhaling through the nose, do all the contractions:

Contract your anterior and posterior openings.

Squeeze the ball with your knees.

Squeeze the balls with your fingers.

Press your tongue to your palate (close your mouth and clench your teeth).

Contract your nostrils.

Your eyes look upward, open (don't contract your forehead; feel as if all the muscles are pulling upward in the direction of your eyes).

Relaxation (inhaling)

Inhale slowly through your nose, fill your lungs with air right into the abdominal cavity, and relax all the contractions.

The movements flow harmoniously.

Repetition

Repeat the relaxation and contraction using the slow technique about 10 times.

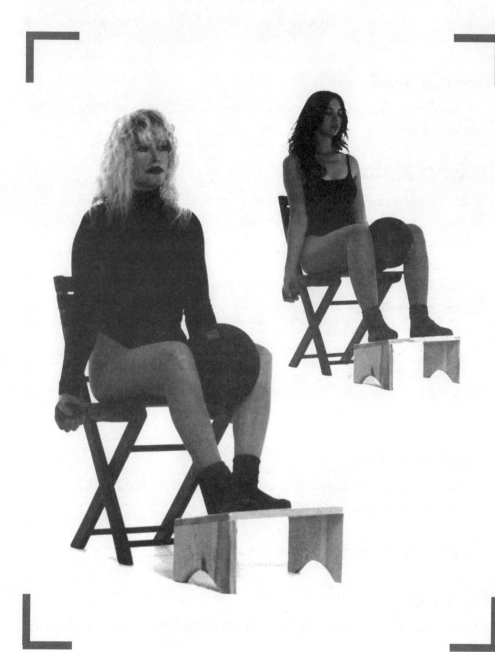

Exercise number 2 - performed sitting on a chair:
Sit upright on a chair, feet on a footrest, knees holding a ball, arms straight out at your sides, each hand holding a ball. (See picture.)

Relaxation (inhaling)

Inhale slowly through your nose, and fill your lungs with air right into the abdominal cavity.

Contraction (exhaling)

Suck your abdomen inward and upward and exhale through your mouth.

When your abdomen is squeezed inward, close your mouth and continue exhaling through your nose.

While exhaling through the nose, do all the contractions:

Contract your anterior and posterior openings.

Squeeze the ball with your knees.

Squeeze the balls with your fingers.

Press your tongue to your palate (close your mouth and clench your teeth).

Contract your nostrils.

Your eyes look upward, open (don't contract your forehead; feel as if all the muscles are pulling upward in the direction of your eyes).

Relaxation (inhaling)

Inhale slowly through your nose, fill your lungs with air right into the abdominal cavity, and relax all the contractions.

The movements flow harmoniously.

Repetition

Repeat the relaxation and contraction using the slow technique about 10 times.

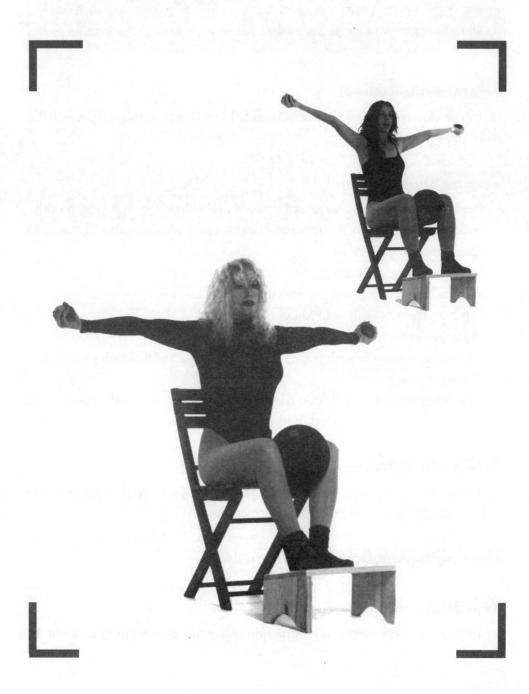

Exercise number 3 - performed sitting on a chair:

Sit upright on a chair, feet on a footrest, knees holding a ball, arms straight up above your head, each hand holding a ball. (See picture.)

Relaxation (inhaling)

Inhale slowly through your nose, and fill your lungs with air right into the abdominal cavity.

Contraction (exhaling)

Suck your abdomen inward and upward and exhale through your mouth.

When your abdomen is squeezed inward, close your mouth and continue exhaling through your nose.

While exhaling through the nose, do all the contractions:

Contract your anterior and posterior openings.

Squeeze the ball with your knees.

Squeeze the balls with your fingers.

Press your tongue to your palate (close your mouth and clench your teeth).

Contract your nostrils.

Your eyes look upward, open (don't contract your forehead; feel as if all the muscles are pulling upward in the direction of your eyes).

Relaxation (inhaling)

Inhale slowly through your nose, fill your lungs with air right into the abdominal cavity, and relax all the contractions.

The movements flow harmoniously.

Repetition

Repeat the relaxation and contraction using the slow technique about 10 times.

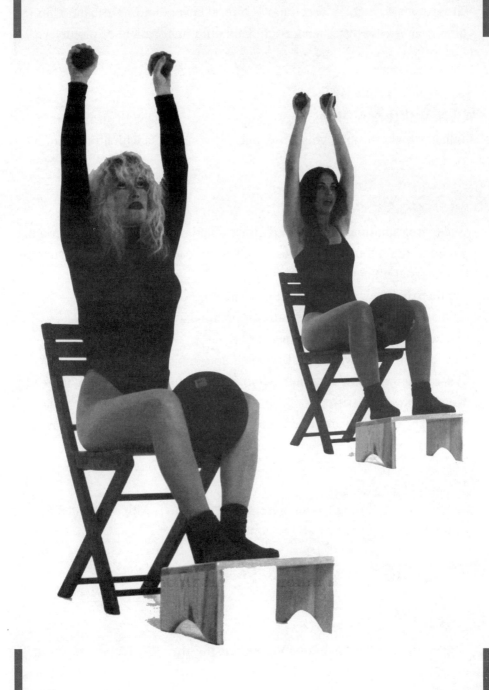

Exercise number 4 - performed sitting on a chair:

Sit upright on a chair, feet on a footrest the same height as your chair (or on another chair), knees holding a ball, arms straight down at your sides, each hand holding a ball. (See picture.)

Relaxation (inhaling)

Inhale slowly through your nose, and fill your lungs with air right into the abdominal cavity.

Contraction (exhaling)

Suck your abdomen inward and upward and exhale through your mouth.

When your abdomen is squeezed inward, close your mouth and continue exhaling through your nose.

While exhaling through the nose, do all the contractions:

Contract your anterior and posterior openings.

Squeeze the ball with your knees.

Squeeze the balls with your fingers.

Press your tongue to your palate (close your mouth and clench your teeth).

Contract your nostrils.

Your eyes look upward, open (don't contract your forehead; feel as if all the muscles are pulling upward in the direction of your eyes).

Relaxation (inhaling)

Inhale slowly through your nose, fill your lungs with air right into the abdominal cavity, and relax all the contractions.

The movements flow harmoniously.

Repetition

Repeat the relaxation and contraction using the slow technique about 10 times.

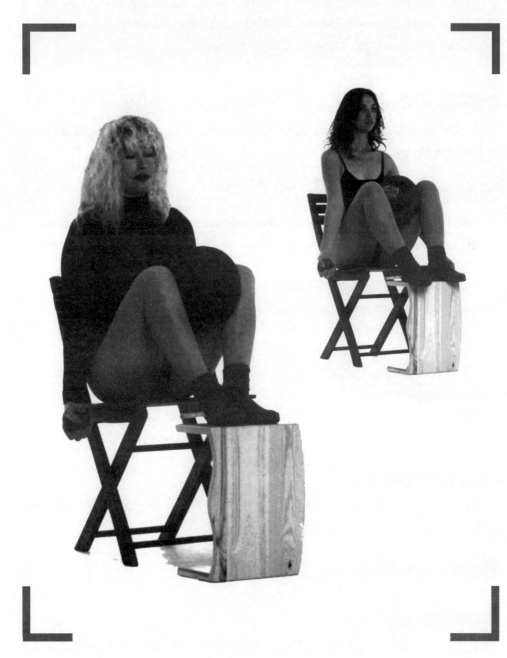

> ## Exercise number 5 - performed sitting on a chair:
> Sit upright on a chair, feet on a footrest the same height as your chair (or on another chair), knees holding a ball, arms straight out at your sides, each hand holding a ball. (See picture.)

Relaxation (inhaling)

Inhale slowly through your nose, and fill your lungs with air right into the abdominal cavity.

Contraction (exhaling)

Suck your abdomen inward and upward and exhale through your mouth.

When your abdomen is squeezed inward, close your mouth and continue exhaling through your nose.

While exhaling through the nose, do all the contractions:

Contract your anterior and posterior openings.

Squeeze the ball with your knees.

Squeeze the balls with your fingers.

Press your tongue to your palate (close your mouth and clench your teeth).

Contract your nostrils.

Your eyes look upward, open (don't contract your forehead; feel as if all the muscles are pulling upward in the direction of your eyes).

Relaxation (inhaling)

Inhale slowly through your nose, fill your lungs with air right into the abdominal cavity, and relax all the contractions.

The movements flow harmoniously.

Repetition

Repeat the relaxation and contraction using the slow technique about 10 times.

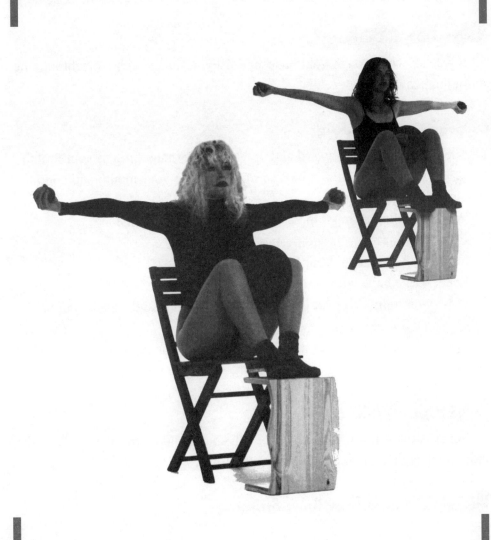

Exercise number 6 - performed sitting on a chair:

Sit upright on a chair, feet on a footrest the same height as your chair (or on another chair), knees holding a ball, arms straight up above your head, each hand holding a ball. (See picture.)

Relaxation (inhaling)

Inhale slowly through your nose, and fill your lungs with air right into the abdominal cavity.

Contraction (exhaling)

Suck your abdomen inward and upward and exhale through your mouth.

When your abdomen is squeezed inward, close your mouth and continue exhaling through your nose.

While exhaling through the nose, do all the contractions:

Contract your anterior and posterior openings.

Squeeze the ball with your knees.

Squeeze the balls with your fingers.

Press your tongue to your palate (close your mouth and clench your teeth).

Contract your nostrils.

Your eyes look upward, open (don't contract your forehead; feel as if all the muscles are pulling upward in the direction of your eyes).

Relaxation (inhaling)

Inhale slowly through your nose, fill your lungs with air right into the abdominal cavity, and relax all the contractions.

The movements flow harmoniously.

Repetition

Repeat the relaxation and contraction using the slow technique about 10 times.

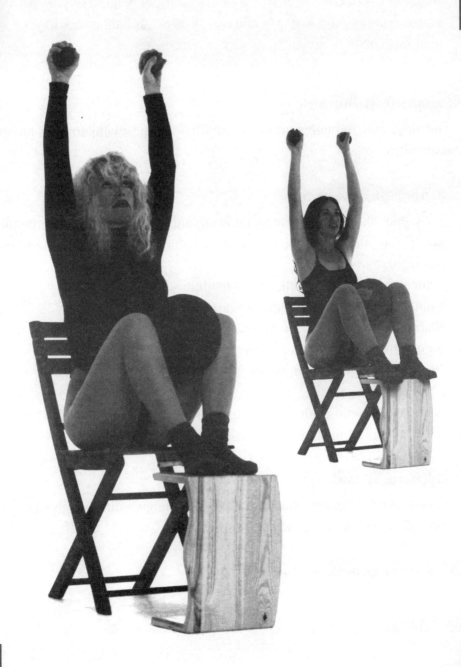

Exercise number 7 - performed sitting on a chair:

Sit upright on a chair, legs straight out in front of you, knees holding a ball, arms straight down at your sides, each hand holding a ball. (See picture.)

Relaxation (inhaling)

Inhale slowly through your nose, and fill your lungs with air right into the abdominal cavity.

Contraction (exhaling)

Suck your abdomen inward and upward and exhale through your mouth.

When your abdomen is squeezed inward, close your mouth and continue exhaling through your nose.

While exhaling through the nose, do all the contractions:

Contract your anterior and posterior openings.

Squeeze the ball with your knees.

Squeeze the balls with your fingers.

Press your tongue to your palate (close your mouth and clench your teeth).

Contract your nostrils.

Your eyes look upward, open (don't contract your forehead; feel as if all the muscles are pulling upward in the direction of your eyes).

Relaxation (inhaling)

Inhale slowly through your nose, fill your lungs with air right into the abdominal cavity, and relax all the contractions.

The movements flow harmoniously.

Repetition

Repeat the relaxation and contraction using the slow technique about 10 times.

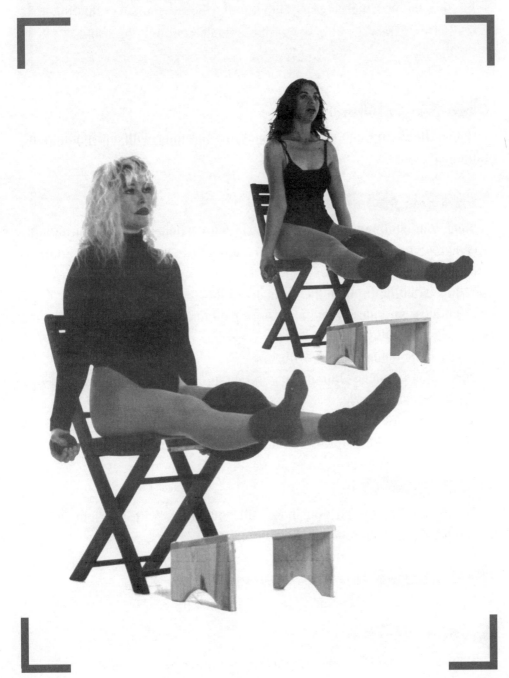

Exercise number 8 - performed sitting on a chair:

Sit upright on a chair, legs straight out in front of you, knees holding a ball, arms straight out at your sides, each hand holding a ball. (See picture.)

Relaxation (inhaling)

Inhale slowly through your nose, and fill your lungs with air right into the abdominal cavity.

Contraction (exhaling)

Suck your abdomen inward and upward and exhale through your mouth.

When your abdomen is squeezed inward, close your mouth and continue exhaling through your nose.

While exhaling through the nose, do all the contractions:

Contract your anterior and posterior openings.

Squeeze the ball with your knees.

Squeeze the balls with your fingers.

Press your tongue to your palate (close your mouth and clench your teeth).

Contract your nostrils.

Your eyes look upward, open (don't contract your forehead; feel as if all the muscles are pulling upward in the direction of your eyes).

Relaxation (inhaling)

Inhale slowly through your nose, fill your lungs with air right into the abdominal cavity, and relax all the contractions.

The movements flow harmoniously.

Repetition

Repeat the relaxation and contraction using the slow technique about 10 times.

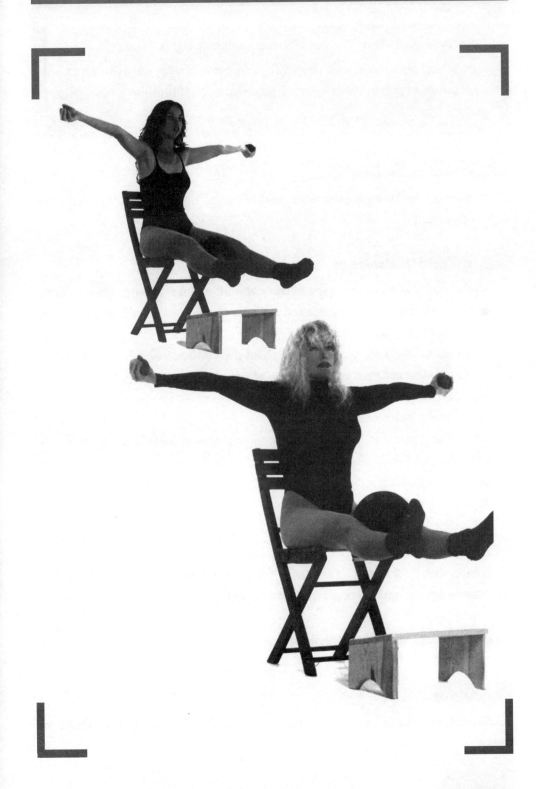

Exercise number 9 - performed sitting on a chair:

Sit upright on a chair, legs straight out in front of you, knees holding a ball, arms straight up above your head, each hand holding a ball. (See picture.)

Relaxation (inhaling)

Inhale slowly through your nose, and fill your lungs with air right into the abdominal cavity.

Contraction (exhaling)

Suck your abdomen inward and upward and exhale through your mouth.

When your abdomen is squeezed inward, close your mouth and continue exhaling through your nose.

While exhaling through the nose, do all the contractions:

Contract your anterior and posterior openings.

Squeeze the ball with your knees.

Squeeze the balls with your fingers.

Press your tongue to your palate (close your mouth and clench your teeth).

Contract your nostrils.

Your eyes look upward, open (don't contract your forehead; feel as if all the muscles are pulling upward in the direction of your eyes).

Relaxation (inhaling)

Inhale slowly through your nose, fill your lungs with air right into the abdominal cavity, and relax all the contractions.

The movements flow harmoniously.

Repetition

Repeat the relaxation and contraction using the slow technique about 10 times.

Repeat exercises 1-15 lying on your back, using the slow technique, five times.
Repeat the same exercises using the slow asymmetrical technique twice - once on the right side, and once on the left.

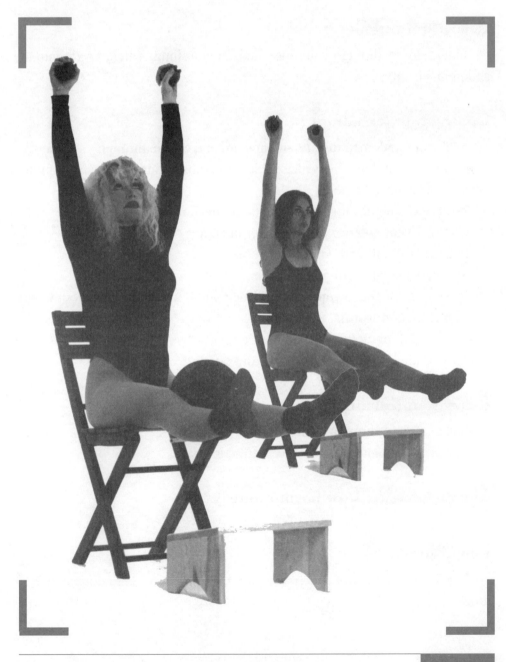

Exercise number 10 - performed sitting on a chair:
Sit upright on a chair, legs straight out in front of you, feet holding a ball, arms straight down at your sides, each hand holding a ball. (See picture.)

Relaxation (inhaling)

Inhale slowly through your nose, and fill your lungs with air right into the abdominal cavity.

Contraction (exhaling)

Suck your abdomen inward and upward and exhale through your mouth.

When your abdomen is squeezed inward, close your mouth and continue exhaling through your nose.

While exhaling through the nose, do all the contractions:

Contract your anterior and posterior openings.

Squeeze the ball with your feet.

Squeeze the balls with your fingers.

Press your tongue to your palate (close your mouth and clench your teeth).

Contract your nostrils.

Your eyes look upward, open (don't contract your forehead; feel as if all the muscles are pulling upward in the direction of your eyes).

Relaxation (inhaling)

Inhale slowly through your nose, fill your lungs with air right into the abdominal cavity, and relax all the contractions.

The movements flow harmoniously.

Repetition

Repeat the relaxation and contraction using the slow technique about 10 times.

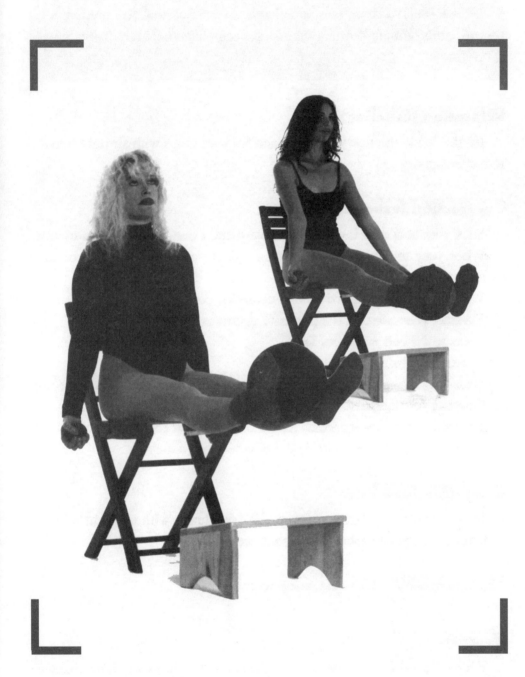

Exercise number 11 - performed sitting on a chair:

Sit upright on a chair, legs straight out in front of you, feet holding a ball, arms straight out at your sides, each hand holding a ball. (See picture.)

Relaxation (inhaling)

Inhale slowly through your nose, and fill your lungs with air right into the abdominal cavity.

Contraction (exhaling)

Suck your abdomen inward and upward and exhale through your mouth.

When your abdomen is squeezed inward, close your mouth and continue exhaling through your nose.

While exhaling through the nose, do all the contractions:

Contract your anterior and posterior openings.

Squeeze the ball with your feet.

Squeeze the balls with your fingers.

Press your tongue to your palate (close your mouth and clench your teeth).

Contract your nostrils.

Your eyes look upward, open (don't contract your forehead; feel as if all the muscles are pulling upward in the direction of your eyes).

Relaxation (inhaling)

Inhale slowly through your nose, fill your lungs with air right into the abdominal cavity, and relax all the contractions.

The movements flow harmoniously.

Repetition

Repeat the relaxation and contraction using the slow technique about 10 times.

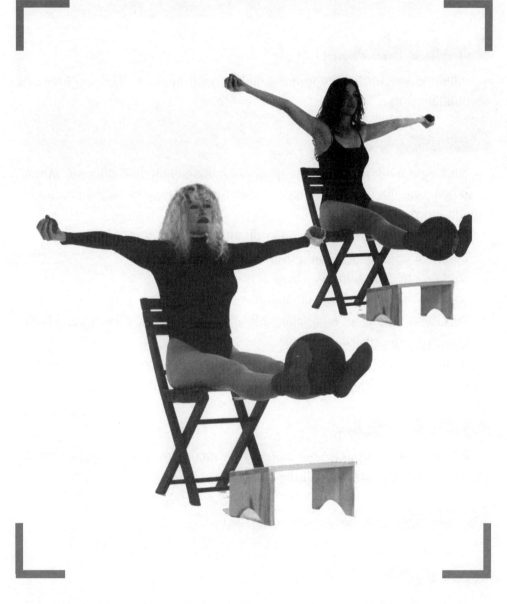

Exercise number 12 - performed sitting on a chair:

Sit upright on a chair, legs straight out in front of you, feet holding a ball, arms straight up above your head, each hand holding a ball. (See picture.)

Relaxation (inhaling)

Inhale slowly through your nose, and fill your lungs with air right into the abdominal cavity.

Contraction (exhaling)

Suck your abdomen inward and upward and exhale through your mouth.

When your abdomen is squeezed inward, close your mouth and continue exhaling through your nose.

While exhaling through the nose, do all the contractions:

Contract your anterior and posterior openings.

Squeeze the ball with your feet.

Squeeze the balls with your fingers.

Press your tongue to your palate (close your mouth and clench your teeth).

Contract your nostrils.

Your eyes look upward, open (don't contract your forehead; feel as if all the muscles are pulling upward in the direction of your eyes).

Relaxation (inhaling)

Inhale slowly through your nose, fill your lungs with air right into the abdominal cavity, and relax all the contractions.

The movements flow harmoniously.

Repetition

Repeat the relaxation and contraction using the slow technique about 10 times.

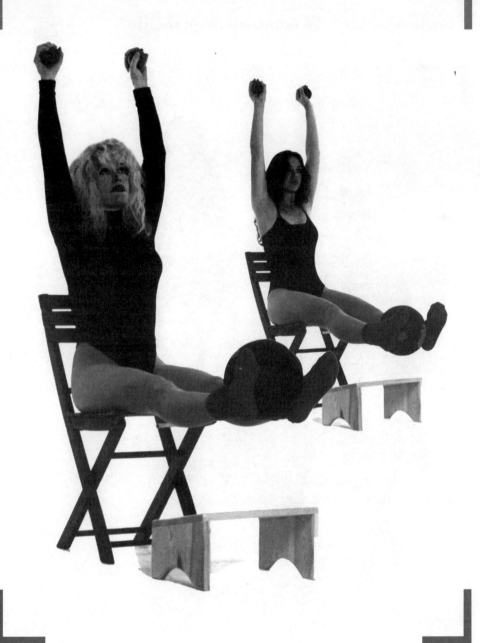

Alternative method: Women who find it difficult to hold their legs straight out in front of them for exercises 7-12 can use a support for their legs. (See pictures.)

Exercise number   7 (alternative method):

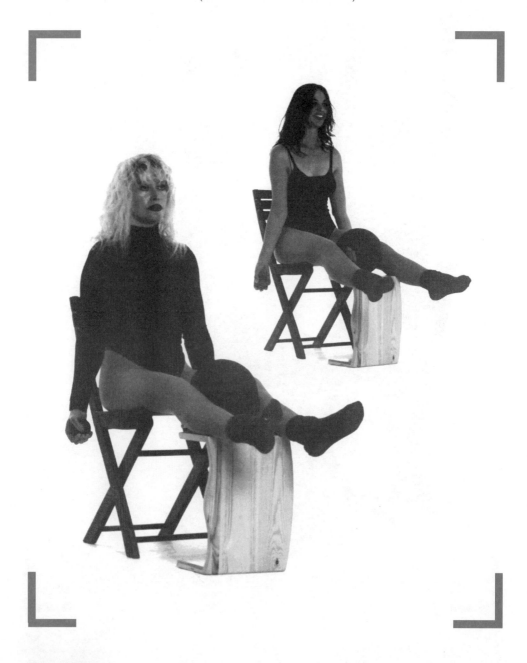

Exercise number   8 (alternative method):

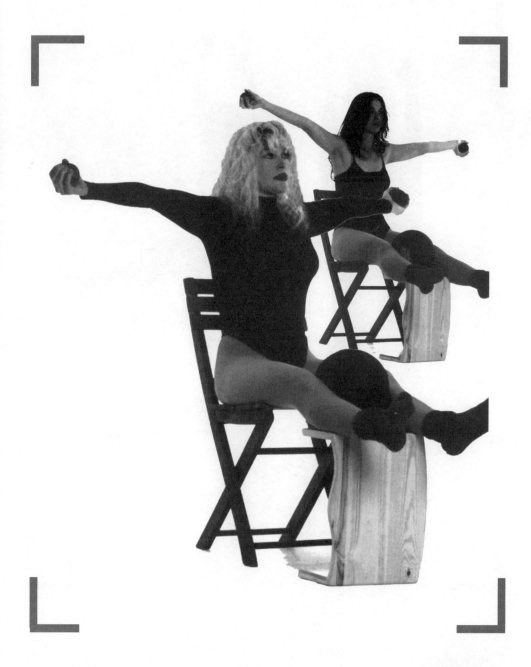

Exercise number   9 (alternative method):

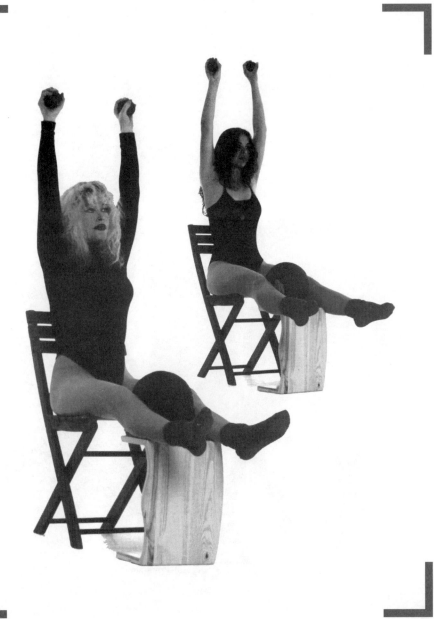

Exercises for Women

Exercise number   10 (alternative method):

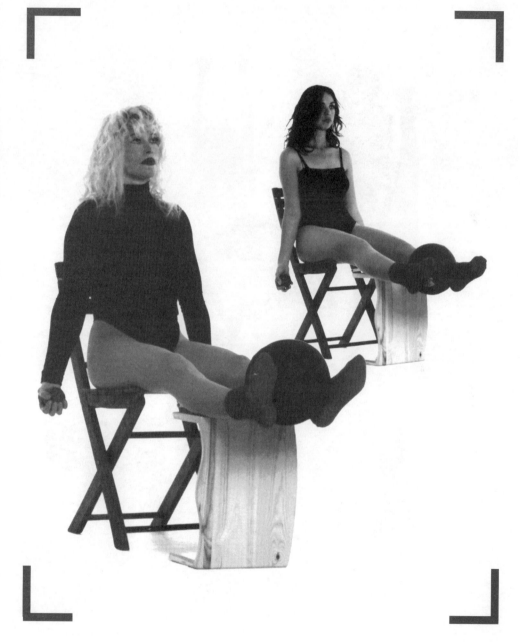

Exercise number   11 (alternative method):

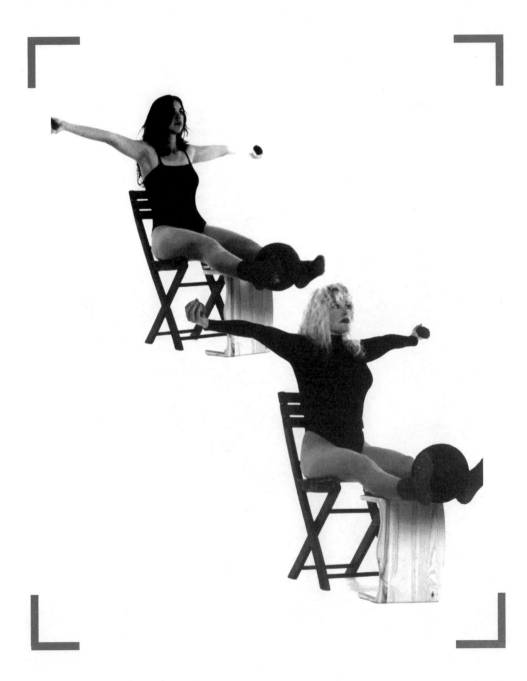

Exercises for Women

Exercise number   12 (alternative method):

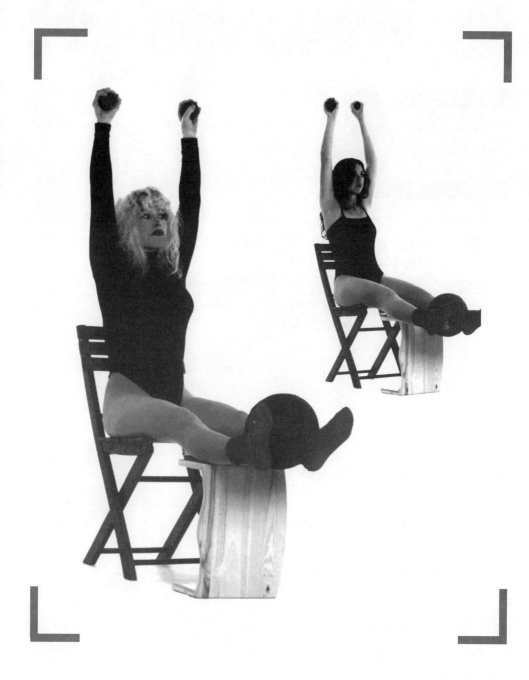

Exercise number 13 - performed sitting on a chair:

Sit upright on a chair, knees bent, feet on a footrest the same height as your chair (or on another chair), knees holding a ball, arms straight out in front of you, holding a ball. (See picture.)

Relaxation (inhaling)

Inhale slowly through your nose, and fill your lungs with air right into the abdominal cavity.

Contraction (exhaling)

Suck your abdomen inward and upward and exhale through your mouth.

When your abdomen is squeezed inward, close your mouth and continue exhaling through your nose.

While exhaling through the nose, do all the contractions:

Contract your anterior and posterior openings.

Squeeze the ball with your knees.

Squeeze the ball with your hands.

Press your tongue to your palate (close your mouth and clench your teeth).

Contract your nostrils.

Your eyes look upward, open (don't contract your forehead; feel as if all the muscles are pulling upward in the direction of your eyes).

Relaxation (inhaling)

Inhale slowly through your nose, fill your lungs with air right into the abdominal cavity, and relax all the contractions.

The movements flow harmoniously.

Repetition

Repeat the relaxation and contraction using the slow technique about 10 times.

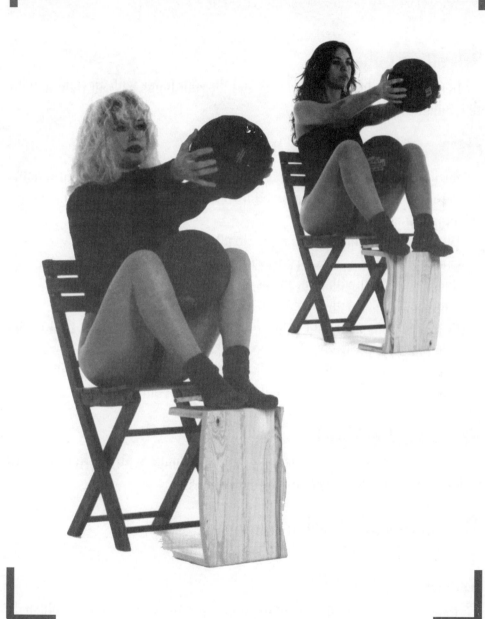

Exercise number 14 - performed sitting on a chair:

Sit upright on a chair, knees bent, feet on a footrest the same height as your chair (or on another chair), knees holding a ball, arms straight up above your head, holding a ball. (See picture.)

Relaxation (inhaling)

Inhale slowly through your nose, and fill your lungs with air right into the abdominal cavity.

Contraction (exhaling)

Suck your abdomen inward and upward and exhale through your mouth.

When your abdomen is squeezed inward, close your mouth and continue exhaling through your nose.

While exhaling through the nose, do all the contractions:

Contract your anterior and posterior openings.

Squeeze the ball with your knees.

Squeeze the ball with your hands.

Press your tongue to your palate (close your mouth and clench your teeth).

Contract your nostrils.

Your eyes look upward, open (don't contract your forehead; feel as if all the muscles are pulling upward in the direction of your eyes).

Relaxation (inhaling)

Inhale slowly through your nose, fill your lungs with air right into the abdominal cavity, and relax all the contractions.

The movements flow harmoniously.

Repetition

Repeat the relaxation and contraction using the slow technique about 10 times.

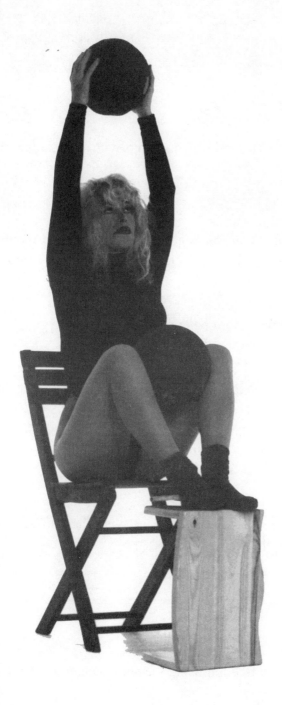
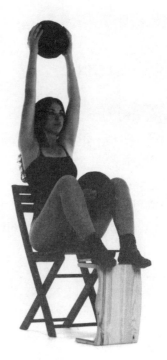

Exercise number 15 - performed sitting on a chair:

Sit upright on a chair, legs straight out in front of you, on a footrest the same height as your chair (or on another chair), knees holding a ball, arms straight out in front of you, holding a ball. (See picture.)

Relaxation (inhaling)

Inhale slowly through your nose, and fill your lungs with air right into the abdominal cavity.

Contraction (exhaling)

Suck your abdomen inward and upward and exhale through your mouth.

When your abdomen is squeezed inward, close your mouth and continue exhaling through your nose.

While exhaling through the nose, do all the contractions:

Contract your anterior and posterior openings.

Squeeze the ball with your knees.

Squeeze the ball with your hands.

Press your tongue to your palate (close your mouth and clench your teeth).

Contract your nostrils.

Your eyes look upward, open (don't contract your forehead; feel as if all the muscles are pulling upward in the direction of your eyes).

Relaxation (inhaling)

Inhale slowly through your nose, fill your lungs with air right into the abdominal cavity, and relax all the contractions.

The movements flow harmoniously.

Repetition

Repeat the relaxation and contraction using the slow technique about 10 times.

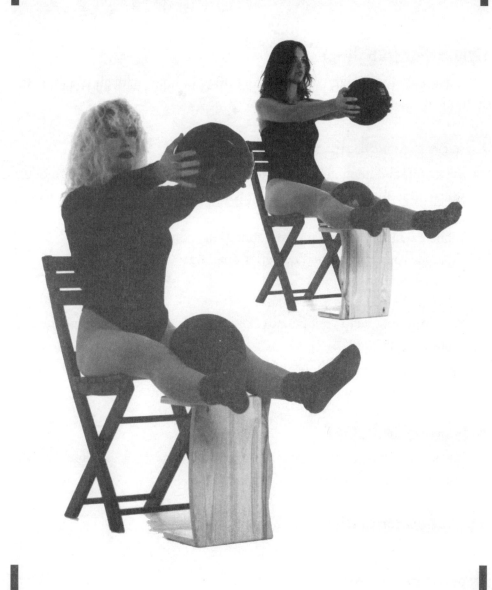

Exercise number 16 - performed sitting on a chair:

Sit upright on a chair, legs straight out in front of you, on a footrest the same height as your chair (or on another chair), knees holding a ball, arms straight up above your head, holding a ball. (See picture.)

Relaxation (inhaling)

Inhale slowly through your nose, and fill your lungs with air right into the abdominal cavity.

Contraction (exhaling)

Suck your abdomen inward and upward and exhale through your mouth.

When your abdomen is squeezed inward, close your mouth and continue exhaling through your nose.

While exhaling through the nose, do all the contractions:

Contract your anterior and posterior openings.

Squeeze the ball with your knees.

Squeeze the ball with your hands.

Press your tongue to your palate (close your mouth and clench your teeth).

Contract your nostrils.

Your eyes look upward, open (don't contract your forehead; feel as if all the muscles are pulling upward in the direction of your eyes).

Relaxation (inhaling)

Inhale slowly through your nose, fill your lungs with air right into the abdominal cavity, and relax all the contractions.

The movements flow harmoniously.

Repetition

Repeat the relaxation and contraction using the slow technique about 10 times.

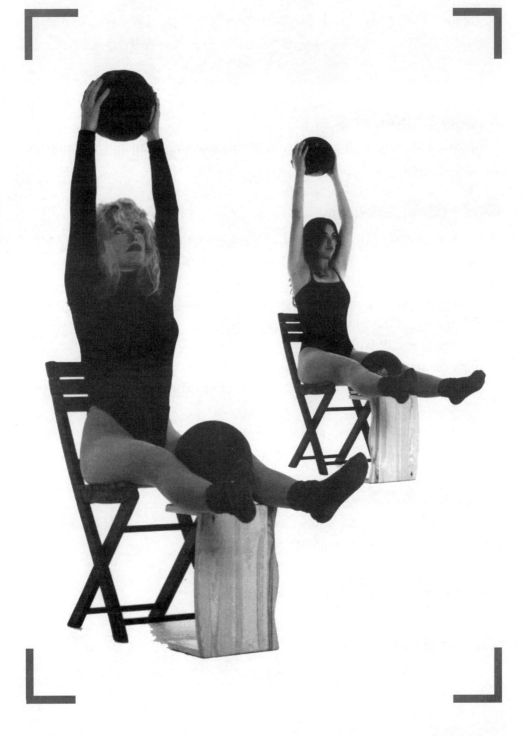

Exercise number 17 - performed sitting on a chair:

Sit upright on a chair, legs straight out in front of you, on a footrest the same height as your chair (or on another chair), feet holding a ball, arms straight out in front of you, holding a ball. (See picture.)

Relaxation (inhaling)

Inhale slowly through your nose, and fill your lungs with air right into the abdominal cavity.

Contraction (exhaling)

Suck your abdomen inward and upward and exhale through your mouth.

When your abdomen is squeezed inward, close your mouth and continue exhaling through your nose.

While exhaling through the nose, do all the contractions:

Contract your anterior and posterior openings.

Squeeze the ball with your feet.

Squeeze the ball with your hands.

Press your tongue to your palate (close your mouth and clench your teeth).

Contract your nostrils.

Your eyes look upward, open (don't contract your forehead; feel as if all the muscles are pulling upward in the direction of your eyes).

Relaxation (inhaling)

Inhale slowly through your nose, fill your lungs with air right into the abdominal cavity, and relax all the contractions.

The movements flow harmoniously.

Repetition

Repeat the relaxation and contraction using the slow technique about 10 times.

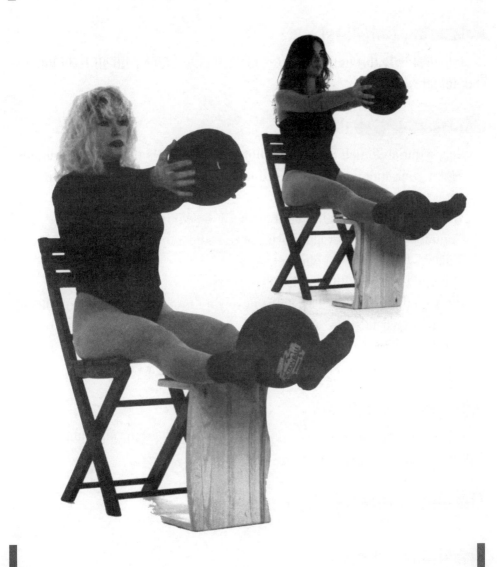

Exercise number 18 - performed sitting on a chair:

Sit upright on a chair, legs straight out in front of you, on a footrest the same height as your chair (or on another chair), feet holding a ball, arms straight up above your head, holding a ball. (See picture.)

Relaxation (inhaling)

Inhale slowly through your nose, and fill your lungs with air right into the abdominal cavity.

Contraction (exhaling)

Suck your abdomen inward and upward and exhale through your mouth.

When your abdomen is squeezed inward, close your mouth and continue exhaling through your nose.

While exhaling through the nose, do all the contractions:

Contract your anterior and posterior openings.

Squeeze the ball with your feet.

Squeeze the ball with your hands.

Press your tongue to your palate (close your mouth and clench your teeth).

Contract your nostrils.

Your eyes look upward, open (don't contract your forehead; feel as if all the muscles are pulling upward in the direction of your eyes).

Relaxation (inhaling)

Inhale slowly through your nose, fill your lungs with air right into the abdominal cavity, and relax all the contractions.

The movements flow harmoniously.

Repetition

Repeat the relaxation and contraction using the slow technique about 10 times.

Repeat exercises 1-15 lying on your back, using the slow technique, five times.
Repeat the same exercises using the slow asymmetrical technique twice - once on the right side, and once on the left.

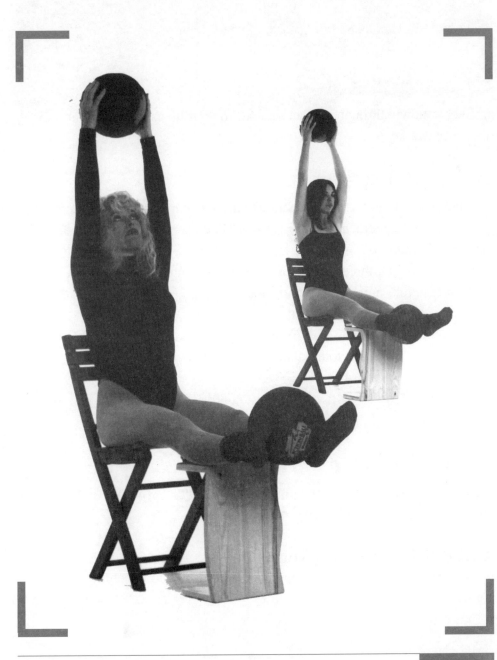

Second week: seventh day

Exercise number 1 - performed standing up with one large and two small balls:

Stand upright, knees holding a ball, arms straight down at the sides of your body, each hand holding a ball. (See picture.)

Relaxation (inhaling)

Inhale slowly through your nose, and fill your lungs with air right into the abdominal cavity.

Contraction (exhaling)

Suck your abdomen inward and upward and exhale through your mouth.

When your abdomen is squeezed inward, close your mouth and continue exhaling through your nose.

While exhaling through the nose, do all the contractions:

Contract your anterior and posterior openings.

Squeeze the ball with your knees.

Squeeze the balls with your fingers.

Press your tongue to your palate (close your mouth and clench your teeth).

Contract your nostrils.

Your eyes look upward, open (don't contract your forehead; feel as if all the muscles are pulling upward in the direction of your eyes).

Relaxation (inhaling)

Inhale slowly through your nose, fill your lungs with air right into the abdominal cavity, and relax all the contractions.

The movements flow harmoniously.

Repetition

Repeat the relaxation and contraction using the slow technique about 10 times.

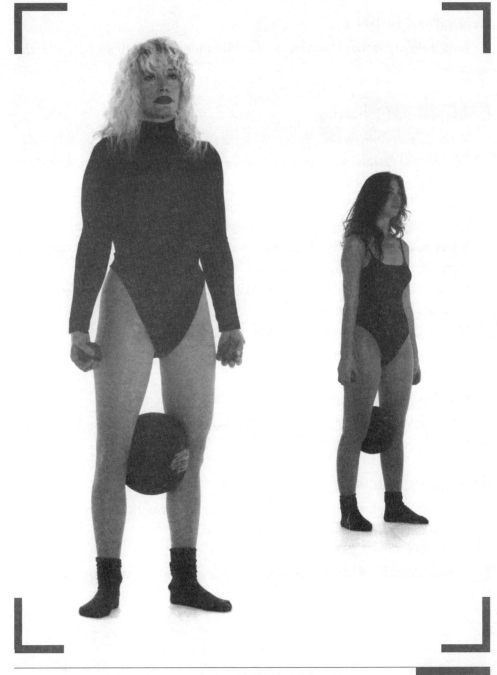

Exercise number 2 - performed standing up:
Stand upright, knees holding a ball, arms straight out at the sides of your body, each hand holding a ball. (See picture.)

Relaxation (inhaling)

Inhale slowly through your nose, and fill your lungs with air right into the abdominal cavity.

Contraction (exhaling)

Suck your abdomen inward and upward and exhale through your mouth.

When your abdomen is squeezed inward, close your mouth and continue exhaling through your nose.

While exhaling through the nose, do all the contractions:

Contract your anterior and posterior openings.

Squeeze the ball with your knees.

Squeeze the balls with your fingers.

Press your tongue to your palate (close your mouth and clench your teeth).

Contract your nostrils.

Your eyes look upward, open (don't contract your forehead; feel as if all the muscles are pulling upward in the direction of your eyes).

Relaxation (inhaling)

Inhale slowly through your nose, fill your lungs with air right into the abdominal cavity, and relax all the contractions.

The movements flow harmoniously.

Repetition

Repeat the relaxation and contraction using the slow technique about 10 times.

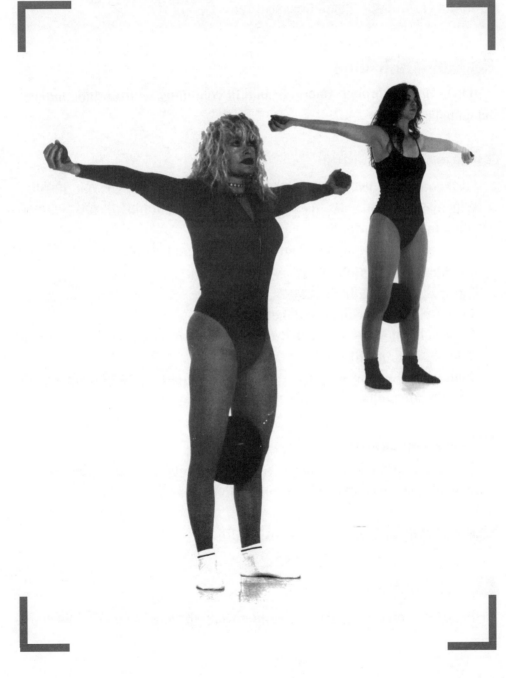

Exercise number 3 - performed standing up:

Stand upright, knees holding a ball, arms straight up above your head, each hand holding a ball. (See picture.)

Relaxation (inhaling)

Inhale slowly through your nose, and fill your lungs with air right into the abdominal cavity.

Contraction (exhaling)

Suck your abdomen inward and upward and exhale through your mouth.

When your abdomen is squeezed inward, close your mouth and continue exhaling through your nose.

While exhaling through the nose, do all the contractions:

Contract your anterior and posterior openings.

Squeeze the ball with your knees.

Squeeze the balls with your fingers.

Press your tongue to your palate (close your mouth and clench your teeth).

Contract your nostrils.

Your eyes look upward, open (don't contract your forehead; feel as if all the muscles are pulling upward in the direction of your eyes).

Relaxation (inhaling)

Inhale slowly through your nose, fill your lungs with air right into the abdominal cavity, and relax all the contractions.

The movements flow harmoniously.

Repetition

Repeat the relaxation and contraction using the slow technique about 10 times.

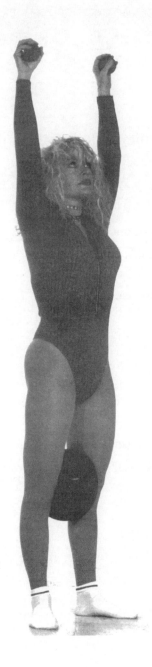
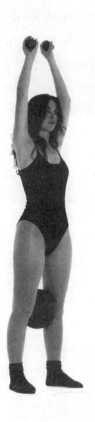

Exercise number 4 - performed standing up:
Stand upright, knees holding a ball, arms straight down at the sides of your body, each hand holding a ball. During the contraction, stand on your tiptoes; during relaxation, stand normally on the soles of your feet. (See picture.)

Relaxation (inhaling)

Inhale slowly through your nose, and fill your lungs with air right into the abdominal cavity.

Contraction (exhaling)

Suck your abdomen inward and upward and exhale through your mouth.

When your abdomen is squeezed inward, close your mouth and continue exhaling through your nose.

While exhaling through the nose, do all the contractions:

Stand on your tiptoes.

Contract your anterior and posterior openings.

Squeeze the ball with your knees.

Squeeze the balls with your fingers.

Press your tongue to your palate (close your mouth and clench your teeth).

Contract your nostrils.

Your eyes look upward, open (don't contract your forehead; feel as if all the muscles are pulling upward in the direction of your eyes).

Relaxation (inhaling)

Stand normally on the soles of your feet.

Inhale slowly through your nose, fill your lungs with air right into the abdominal cavity, and relax all the contractions.

The movements flow harmoniously.

Repetition

Repeat the relaxation and contraction using the slow technique about 10 times.

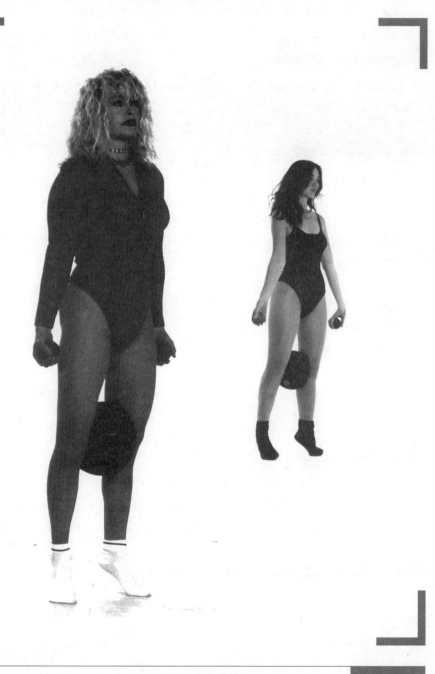

Exercise number 5 - performed standing up:

Stand upright, knees holding a ball, arms straight out at the sides of your body, each hand holding a ball. During the contraction, stand on your tiptoes; during relaxation, stand normally on the soles of your feet. (See picture.)

Relaxation (inhaling)

Inhale slowly through your nose, and fill your lungs with air right into the abdominal cavity.

Contraction (exhaling)

Suck your abdomen inward and upward and exhale through your mouth.

When your abdomen is squeezed inward, close your mouth and continue exhaling through your nose.

While exhaling through the nose, do all the contractions:

Stand on your tiptoes.

Contract your anterior and posterior openings.

Squeeze the ball with your knees.

Squeeze the balls with your fingers.

Press your tongue to your palate (close your mouth and clench your teeth).

Contract your nostrils.

Your eyes look upward, open (don't contract your forehead; feel as if all the muscles are pulling upward in the direction of your eyes).

Relaxation (inhaling)

Stand normally on the soles of your feet.

Inhale slowly through your nose, fill your lungs with air right into the abdominal cavity, and relax all the contractions.

The movements flow harmoniously.

Repetition

Repeat the relaxation and contraction using the slow technique about 10 times.

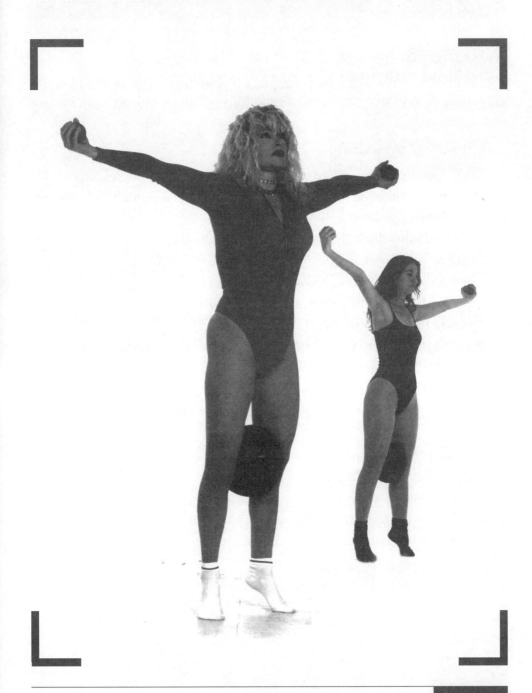

Exercise number 6 - performed standing up:
Stand upright, knees holding a ball, arms straight up above your head, each hand holding a ball. During the contraction, stand on your tiptoes; during relaxation, stand normally on the soles of your feet. (See picture.)

Relaxation (inhaling)

Inhale slowly through your nose, and fill your lungs with air right into the abdominal cavity.

Contraction (exhaling)

Suck your abdomen inward and upward and exhale through your mouth.

When your abdomen is squeezed inward, close your mouth and continue exhaling through your nose.

While exhaling through the nose, do all the contractions:

Stand on your tiptoes.

Contract your anterior and posterior openings.

Squeeze the ball with your knees.

Squeeze the balls with your fingers.

Press your tongue to your palate (close your mouth and clench your teeth).

Contract your nostrils.

Your eyes look upward, open (don't contract your forehead; feel as if all the muscles are pulling upward in the direction of your eyes).

Relaxation (inhaling)

Stand normally on the soles of your feet.

Inhale slowly through your nose, fill your lungs with air right into the abdominal cavity, and relax all the contractions.

The movements flow harmoniously.

Repetition

Repeat the relaxation and contraction using the slow technique about 10 times.

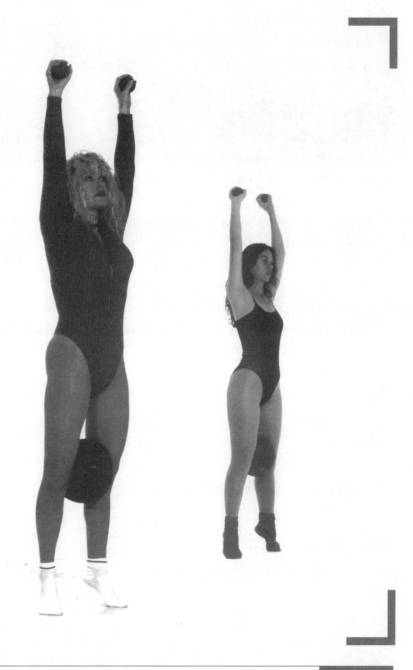

Exercise number 7 - performed standing up:

Stand upright, feet holding a ball, arms straight down at the sides of your body, each hand holding a ball. (See picture.)

Relaxation (inhaling)

Inhale slowly through your nose, and fill your lungs with air right into the abdominal cavity.

Contraction (exhaling)

Suck your abdomen inward and upward and exhale through your mouth.

When your abdomen is squeezed inward, close your mouth and continue exhaling through your nose.

While exhaling through the nose, do all the contractions:

Contract your anterior and posterior openings.

Squeeze the ball with your feet.

Squeeze the balls with your fingers.

Press your tongue to your palate (close your mouth and clench your teeth).

Contract your nostrils.

Your eyes look upward, open (don't contract your forehead; feel as if all the muscles are pulling upward in the direction of your eyes).

Relaxation (inhaling)

Inhale slowly through your nose, fill your lungs with air right into the abdominal cavity, and relax all the contractions.

The movements flow harmoniously.

Repetition

Repeat the relaxation and contraction using the slow technique about 10 times.

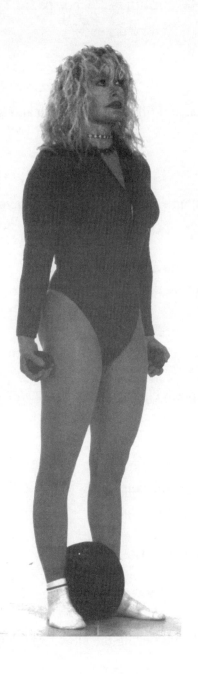
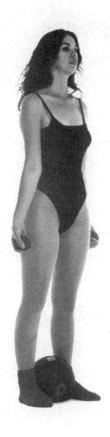

Exercise number 8 - performed standing up:

Stand upright, feet holding a ball, arms straight out at the sides of your body, each hand holding a ball. (See picture.)

Relaxation (inhaling)

Inhale slowly through your nose, and fill your lungs with air right into the abdominal cavity.

Contraction (exhaling)

Suck your abdomen inward and upward and exhale through your mouth.

When your abdomen is squeezed inward, close your mouth and continue exhaling through your nose.

While exhaling through the nose, do all the contractions:

Contract your anterior and posterior openings.

Squeeze the ball with your feet.

Squeeze the balls with your fingers.

Press your tongue to your palate (close your mouth and clench your teeth).

Contract your nostrils.

Your eyes look upward, open (don't contract your forehead; feel as if all the muscles are pulling upward in the direction of your eyes).

Relaxation (inhaling)

Inhale slowly through your nose, fill your lungs with air right into the abdominal cavity, and relax all the contractions.

The movements flow harmoniously.

Repetition

Repeat the relaxation and contraction using the slow technique about 10 times.

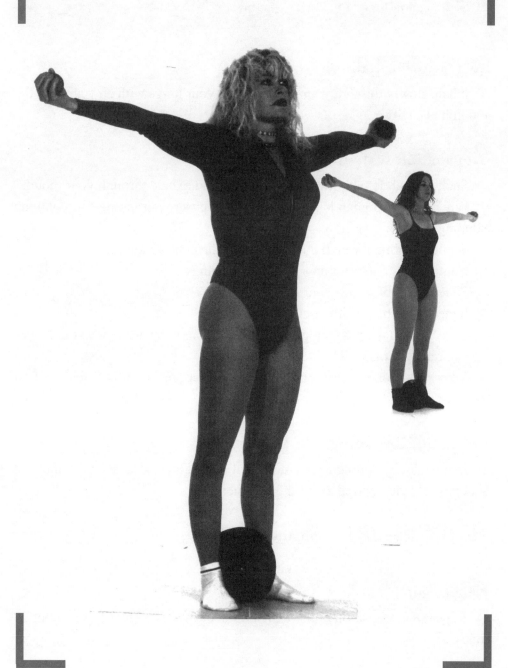

Exercise number 9 - performed standing up:
Stand upright, feet holding a ball, arms straight up above your head, each hand holding a ball. (See picture.)

Relaxation (inhaling)

Inhale slowly through your nose, and fill your lungs with air right into the abdominal cavity.

Contraction (exhaling)

Suck your abdomen inward and upward and exhale through your mouth.

When your abdomen is squeezed inward, close your mouth and continue exhaling through your nose.

While exhaling through the nose, do all the contractions:

Contract your anterior and posterior openings.

Squeeze the ball with your feet.

Squeeze the balls with your fingers.

Press your tongue to your palate (close your mouth and clench your teeth).

Contract your nostrils.

Your eyes look upward, open (don't contract your forehead; feel as if all the muscles are pulling upward in the direction of your eyes).

Relaxation (inhaling)

Inhale slowly through your nose, fill your lungs with air right into the abdominal cavity, and relax all the contractions.

The movements flow harmoniously.

Repetition

Repeat the relaxation and contraction using the slow technique about 10 times.

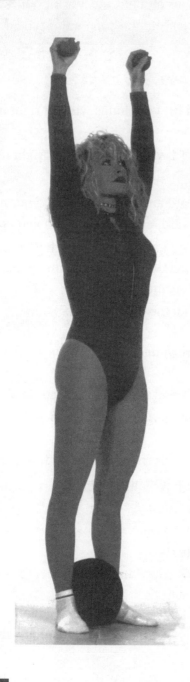

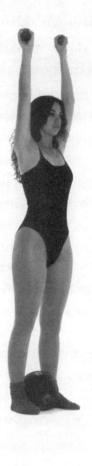

Exercise number 10 - performed standing up:

Stand upright, feet holding a ball, arms straight down at the sides of your body, each hand holding a ball. During the contraction, stand on your tiptoes; during relaxation, stand normally on the soles of your feet. (See picture.)

Relaxation (inhaling)

Inhale slowly through your nose, and fill your lungs with air right into the abdominal cavity.

Contraction (exhaling)

Suck your abdomen inward and upward and exhale through your mouth.

When your abdomen is squeezed inward, close your mouth and continue exhaling through your nose.

While exhaling through the nose, do all the contractions:

Stand on your tiptoes.

Contract your anterior and posterior openings.

Squeeze the ball with your feet.

Squeeze the balls with your fingers.

Press your tongue to your palate (close your mouth and clench your teeth).

Contract your nostrils.

Your eyes look upward, open (don't contract your forehead; feel as if all the muscles are pulling upward in the direction of your eyes).

Relaxation (inhaling)

Stand normally on the soles of your feet.

Inhale slowly through your nose, fill your lungs with air right into the abdominal cavity, and relax all the contractions.

The movements flow harmoniously.

Repetition

Repeat the relaxation and contraction using the slow technique about 10 times.

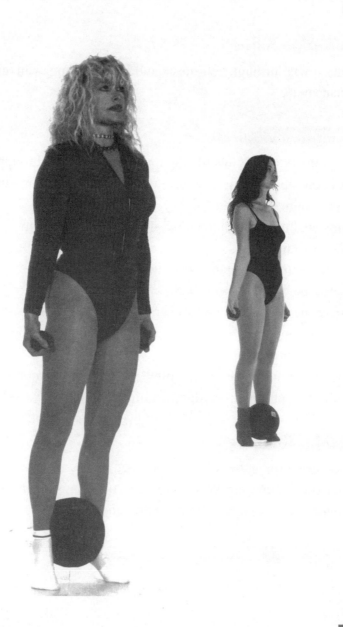

Exercise number 11 - performed standing up:

Stand upright, feet holding a ball, arms straight out at the sides of your body, each hand holding a ball. During the contraction, stand on your tiptoes; during relaxation, stand normally on the soles of your feet. (See picture.)

Relaxation (inhaling)

Inhale slowly through your nose, and fill your lungs with air right into the abdominal cavity.

Contraction (exhaling)

Suck your abdomen inward and upward and exhale through your mouth.

When your abdomen is squeezed inward, close your mouth and continue exhaling through your nose.

While exhaling through the nose, do all the contractions:

Stand on your tiptoes.

Contract your anterior and posterior openings.

Squeeze the ball with your feet.

Squeeze the balls with your fingers.

Press your tongue to your palate (close your mouth and clench your teeth).

Contract your nostrils.

Your eyes look upward, open (don't contract your forehead; feel as if all the muscles are pulling upward in the direction of your eyes).

Relaxation (inhaling)

Stand normally on the soles of your feet.

Inhale slowly through your nose, fill your lungs with air right into the abdominal cavity, and relax all the contractions.

The movements flow harmoniously.

Repetition

Repeat the relaxation and contraction using the slow technique about 10 times.

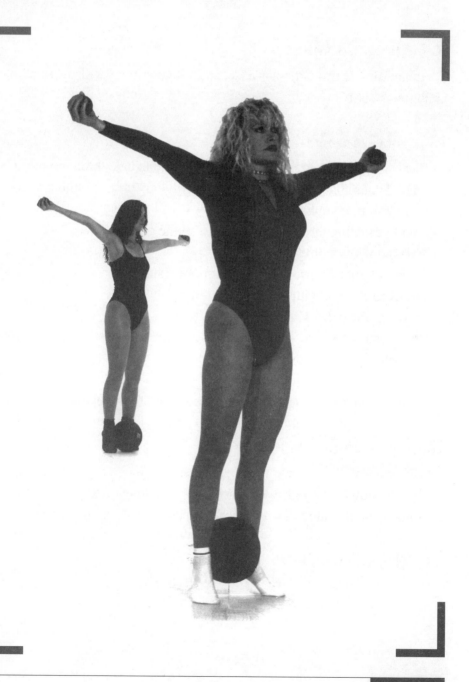

Exercise number 12 - performed standing up:

Stand upright, feet holding a ball, arms straight up above your head, each hand holding a ball. During the contraction, stand on your tiptoes; during relaxation, stand normally on the soles of your feet. (See picture.)

Relaxation (inhaling)

Inhale slowly through your nose, and fill your lungs with air right into the abdominal cavity.

Contraction (exhaling)

Suck your abdomen inward and upward and exhale through your mouth.

When your abdomen is squeezed inward, close your mouth and continue exhaling through your nose.

While exhaling through the nose, do all the contractions:

Stand on your tiptoes.

Contract your anterior and posterior openings.

Squeeze the ball with your feet.

Squeeze the balls with your fingers.

Press your tongue to your palate (close your mouth and clench your teeth).

Contract your nostrils.

Your eyes look upward, open (don't contract your forehead; feel as if all the muscles are pulling upward in the direction of your eyes).

Relaxation (inhaling)

Stand normally on the soles of your feet.

Inhale slowly through your nose, fill your lungs with air right into the abdominal cavity, and relax all the contractions.

The movements flow harmoniously.

Repetition

Repeat the relaxation and contraction using the slow technique about 10 times.

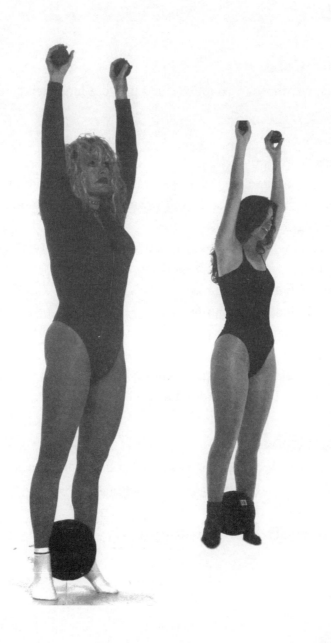

Alternative method for the seventh day of the second week:

Exercise number 1 - performed standing up with two large balls:

Stand upright, knees holding a ball, arms straight out in front of you, holding a ball. (See picture.)

Relaxation (inhaling)

Inhale slowly through your nose, and fill your lungs with air right into the abdominal cavity.

Contraction (exhaling)

Suck your abdomen inward and upward and exhale through your mouth.

When your abdomen is squeezed inward, close your mouth and continue exhaling through your nose.

While exhaling through the nose, do all the contractions:

Contract your anterior and posterior openings.

Squeeze the ball with your knees.

Squeeze the ball with your hands.

Press your tongue to your palate (close your mouth and clench your teeth).

Contract your nostrils.

Your eyes look upward, open (don't contract your forehead; feel as if all the muscles are pulling upward in the direction of your eyes).

Relaxation (inhaling)

Inhale slowly through your nose, fill your lungs with air right into the abdominal cavity, and relax all the contractions.

The movements flow harmoniously.

Repetition

Repeat the relaxation and contraction using the slow technique about 10 times.

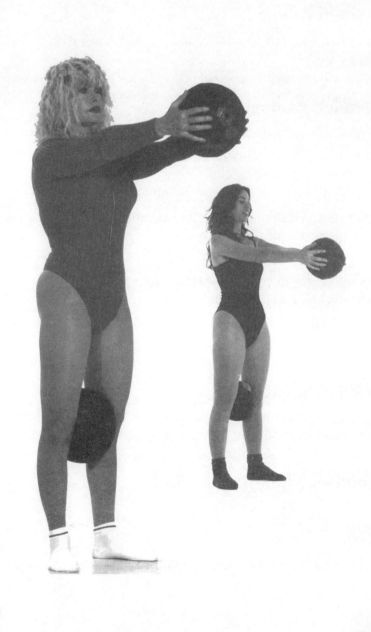

Exercise number 2 - performed standing up with two balls:

upright, knees holding a ball, arms straight up above your head, holding a ball. (See picture.)

Relaxation (inhaling)

Inhale slowly through your nose, and fill your lungs with air right into the abdominal cavity.

Contraction (exhaling)

Suck your abdomen inward and upward and exhale through your mouth.

When your abdomen is squeezed inward, close your mouth and continue exhaling through your nose.

While exhaling through the nose, do all the contractions:

Contract your anterior and posterior openings.

Squeeze the ball with your knees.

Squeeze the ball with your hands.

Press your tongue to your palate (close your mouth and clench your teeth).

Contract your nostrils.

Your eyes look upward, open (don't contract your forehead; feel as if all the muscles are pulling upward in the direction of your eyes).

Relaxation (inhaling)

Inhale slowly through your nose, fill your lungs with air right into the abdominal cavity, and relax all the contractions.

The movements flow harmoniously.

Repetition

Repeat the relaxation and contraction using the slow technique about 10 times.

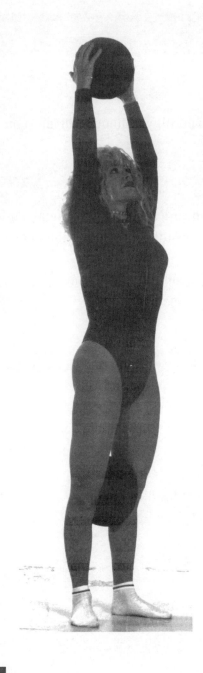
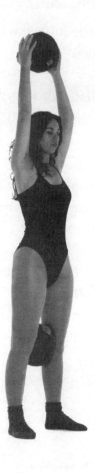

Exercise number 3 - performed standing up with two balls:

Stand upright, knees holding a ball, arms behind your head, holding a ball. (See picture.)

Relaxation (inhaling)

Inhale slowly through your nose, and fill your lungs with air right into the abdominal cavity.

Contraction (exhaling)

Suck your abdomen inward and upward and exhale through your mouth.

When your abdomen is squeezed inward, close your mouth and continue exhaling through your nose.

While exhaling through the nose, do all the contractions:

Contract your anterior and posterior openings.

Squeeze the ball with your knees.

Squeeze the ball with your hands.

Press your tongue to your palate (close your mouth and clench your teeth).

Contract your nostrils.

Your eyes look upward, open (don't contract your forehead; feel as if all the muscles are pulling upward in the direction of your eyes).

Relaxation (inhaling)

Inhale slowly through your nose, fill your lungs with air right into the abdominal cavity, and relax all the contractions.

The movements flow harmoniously.

Repetition

Repeat the relaxation and contraction using the slow technique about 10 times.

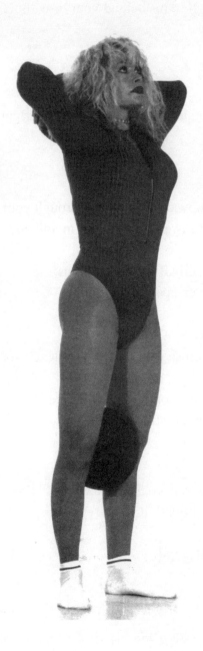
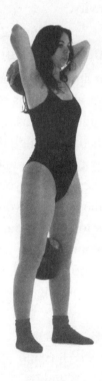

Exercise number 4 - performed standing up with two balls:

Stand upright, knees holding a ball, arms behind your back, holding a ball. (See picture.)

Relaxation (inhaling)

Inhale slowly through your nose, and fill your lungs with air right into the abdominal cavity.

Contraction (exhaling)

Suck your abdomen inward and upward and exhale through your mouth.

When your abdomen is squeezed inward, close your mouth and continue exhaling through your nose.

While exhaling through the nose, do all the contractions:

Contract your anterior and posterior openings.

Squeeze the ball with your knees.

Squeeze the ball with your hands.

Press your tongue to your palate (close your mouth and clench your teeth).

Contract your nostrils.

Your eyes look upward, open (don't contract your forehead; feel as if all the muscles are pulling upward in the direction of your eyes).

Relaxation (inhaling)

Inhale slowly through your nose, fill your lungs with air right into the abdominal cavity, and relax all the contractions.

The movements flow harmoniously.

Repetition

Repeat the relaxation and contraction using the slow technique about 10 times.

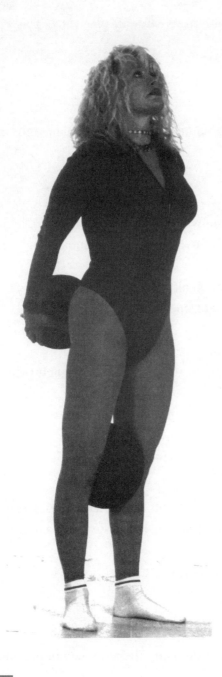
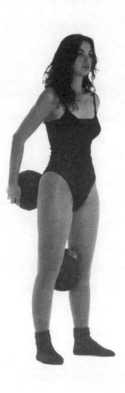

Exercise number 5 - performed standing up with two balls:

Stand upright, feet holding a ball, arms straight out in front of you, holding a ball. (See picture.)

Relaxation (inhaling)

Inhale slowly through your nose, and fill your lungs with air right into the abdominal cavity.

Contraction (exhaling)

Suck your abdomen inward and upward and exhale through your mouth.

When your abdomen is squeezed inward, close your mouth and continue exhaling through your nose.

While exhaling through the nose, do all the contractions:

Contract your anterior and posterior openings.

Squeeze the ball with your feet.

Squeeze the ball with your hands.

Press your tongue to your palate (close your mouth and clench your teeth).

Contract your nostrils.

Your eyes look upward, open (don't contract your forehead; feel as if all the muscles are pulling upward in the direction of your eyes).

Relaxation (inhaling)

Inhale slowly through your nose, fill your lungs with air right into the abdominal cavity, and relax all the contractions.

The movements flow harmoniously.

Repetition

Repeat the relaxation and contraction using the slow technique about 10 times.

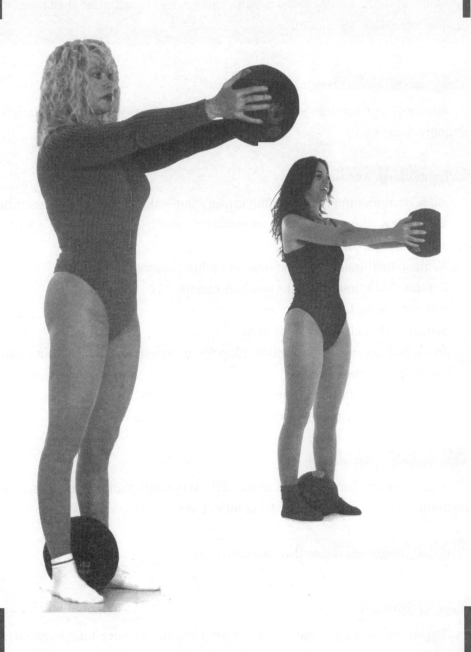

Exercise number 6 - performed standing up with two balls:

Stand upright, feet holding a ball, arms straight up above your head, holding a ball. (See picture.)

Relaxation (inhaling)

Inhale slowly through your nose, and fill your lungs with air right into the abdominal cavity.

Contraction (exhaling)

Suck your abdomen inward and upward and exhale through your mouth.

When your abdomen is squeezed inward, close your mouth and continue exhaling through your nose.

While exhaling through the nose, do all the contractions:

Contract your anterior and posterior openings.

Squeeze the ball with your feet.

Squeeze the ball with your hands.

Press your tongue to your palate (close your mouth and clench your teeth).

Contract your nostrils.

Your eyes look upward, open (don't contract your forehead; feel as if all the muscles are pulling upward in the direction of your eyes).

Relaxation (inhaling)

Inhale slowly through your nose, fill your lungs with air right into the abdominal cavity, and relax all the contractions.

The movements flow harmoniously.

Repetition

Repeat the relaxation and contraction using the slow technique about 10 times.

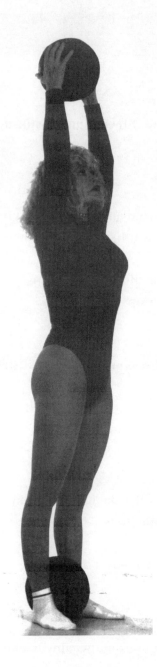
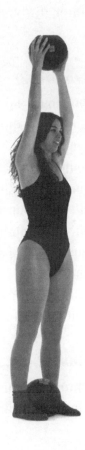

Exercise number 7 - performed standing up
with two balls:

Stand upright, feet holding a ball, arms behind your head, holding a ball. (See picture.)

Relaxation (inhaling)

Inhale slowly through your nose, and fill your lungs with air right into the abdominal cavity.

Contraction (exhaling)

Suck your abdomen inward and upward and exhale through your mouth.

When your abdomen is squeezed inward, close your mouth and continue exhaling through your nose.

While exhaling through the nose, do all the contractions:

Contract your anterior and posterior openings.

Squeeze the ball with your feet.

Squeeze the ball with your hands.

Press your tongue to your palate (close your mouth and clench your teeth).

Contract your nostrils.

Your eyes look upward, open (don't contract your forehead; feel as if all the muscles are pulling upward in the direction of your eyes).

Relaxation (inhaling)

Inhale slowly through your nose, fill your lungs with air right into the abdominal cavity, and relax all the contractions.

The movements flow harmoniously.

Repetition

Repeat the relaxation and contraction using the slow technique about 10 times.

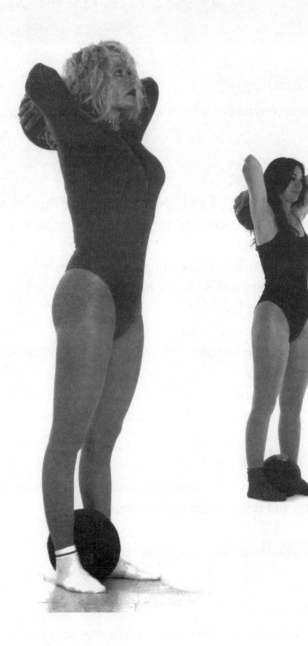

Exercise number 8 - performed standing up with two balls:

Stand upright, feet holding a ball, arms behind your back, holding a ball. (See picture.)

Relaxation (inhaling)

Inhale slowly through your nose, and fill your lungs with air right into the abdominal cavity.

Contraction (exhaling)

Suck your abdomen inward and upward and exhale through your mouth.

When your abdomen is squeezed inward, close your mouth and continue exhaling through your nose.

While exhaling through the nose, do all the contractions:

Contract your anterior and posterior openings.

Squeeze the ball with your feet.

Squeeze the ball with your hands.

Press your tongue to your palate (close your mouth and clench your teeth).

Contract your nostrils.

Your eyes look upward, open (don't contract your forehead; feel as if all the muscles are pulling upward in the direction of your eyes).

Relaxation (inhaling)

Inhale slowly through your nose, fill your lungs with air right into the abdominal cavity, and relax all the contractions.

The movements flow harmoniously.

Repetition

Repeat the relaxation and contraction using the slow technique about 10 times.

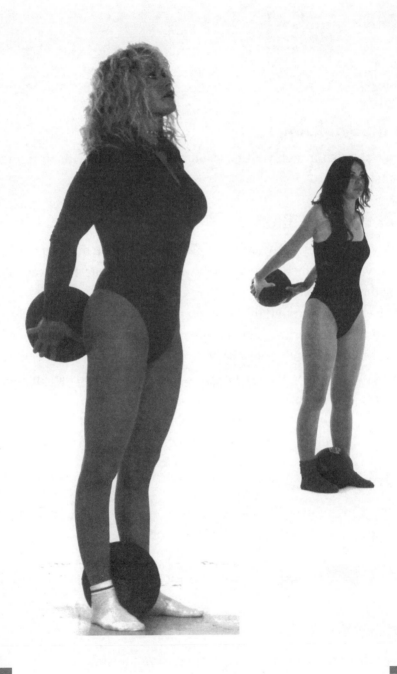

Special exercises (not for every woman)

Exercise number 1:
Lie with your legs over your head, parallel to the floor, knees holding a ball, hands supporting your back. (See picture.)

Relaxation (inhaling)

Inhale slowly through your nose, and fill your lungs with air right into the abdominal cavity.

Contraction (exhaling)

Suck your abdomen inward and upward and exhale through your mouth.

When your abdomen is squeezed inward, close your mouth and continue exhaling through your nose.

While exhaling through the nose, do all the contractions:

Contract your anterior and posterior openings.

Squeeze the ball with your knees.

Press your tongue to your palate (close your mouth and clench your teeth).

Contract your nostrils.

Your eyes look upward, open (don't contract your forehead; feel as if all the muscles are pulling upward in the direction of your eyes).

Relaxation (inhaling)

Inhale slowly through your nose, fill your lungs with air right into the abdominal cavity, and relax all the contractions.

The movements flow harmoniously.

Repetition

Repeat the relaxation and contraction using the slow technique about 10 times.

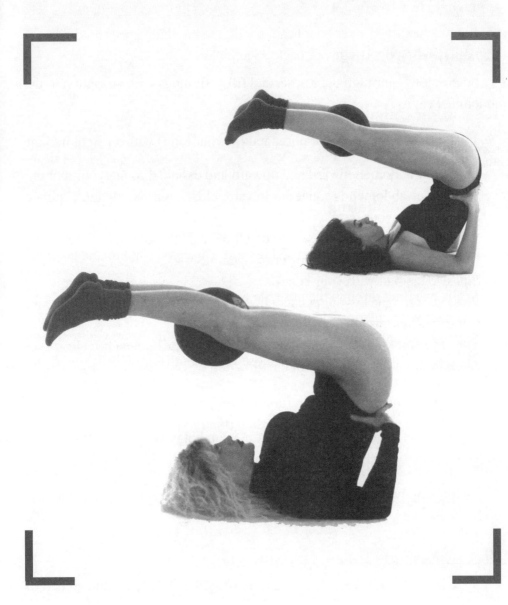

Exercise number 2:

Lie with your legs straight up, knees holding a ball, hands supporting your back. (See picture.)

Relaxation (inhaling)

Inhale slowly through your nose, and fill your lungs with air right into the abdominal cavity.

Contraction (exhaling)

Suck your abdomen inward and upward and exhale through your mouth.

When your abdomen is squeezed inward, close your mouth and continue exhaling through your nose.

While exhaling through the nose, do all the contractions:

Contract your anterior and posterior openings.

Squeeze the ball with your knees.

Press your tongue to your palate (close your mouth and clench your teeth).

Contract your nostrils.

Your eyes look upward, open (don't contract your forehead; feel as if all the muscles are pulling upward in the direction of your eyes).

Relaxation (inhaling)

Inhale slowly through your nose, fill your lungs with air right into the abdominal cavity, and relax all the contractions.

The movements flow harmoniously.

Repetition

Repeat the relaxation and contraction using the slow technique about 10 times.

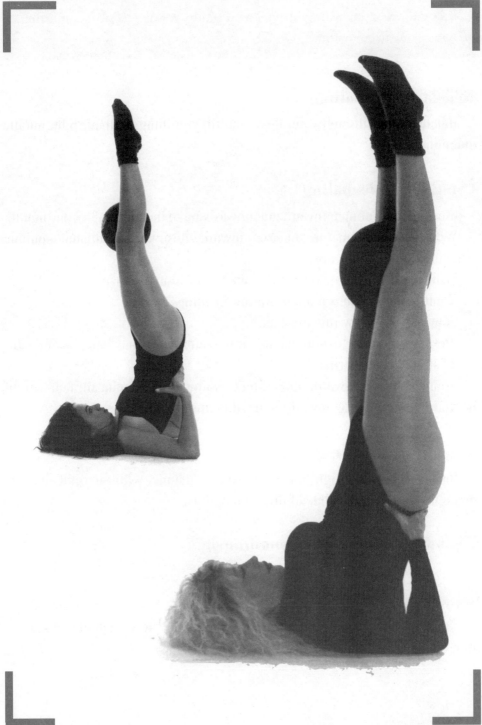

Exercise number 3:

Lie with your legs straight up, feet holding a ball, hands supporting your back. (See picture.)

Relaxation (inhaling)

Inhale slowly through your nose, and fill your lungs with air right into the abdominal cavity.

Contraction (exhaling)

Suck your abdomen inward and upward and exhale through your mouth.

When your abdomen is squeezed inward, close your mouth and continue exhaling through your nose.

While exhaling through the nose, do all the contractions:

Contract your anterior and posterior openings.

Squeeze the ball with your feet.

Press your tongue to your palate (close your mouth and clench your teeth).

Contract your nostrils.

Your eyes look upward, open (don't contract your forehead; feel as if all the muscles are pulling upward in the direction of your eyes).

Relaxation (inhaling)

Inhale slowly through your nose, fill your lungs with air right into the abdominal cavity, and relax all the contractions.

The movements flow harmoniously.

Repetition

Repeat the relaxation and contraction using the slow technique about 10 times.

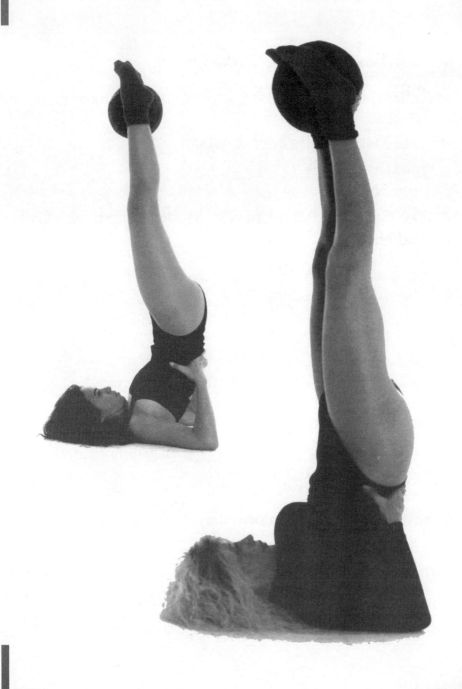

Astrolog ◆ The Quality of Life Series ◆

◆ Exercises for Women - Rivka Gadish
ISBN   965-494-118-X

◆ Thai Massage - Beatrice Avraham
ISBN   965-494-117-1

◆ The Complete Reiki Course - Master Naharo with Gail
Radford
ISBN   965-494-119-8